POWERING
THROUGH
PREGNANCY

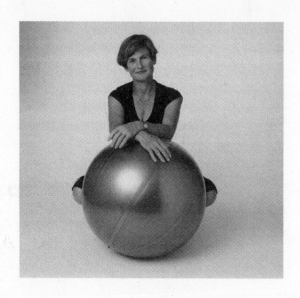

For over 20 years leading obstetric physiotherapist Jane Simons has taught pregnant women how to exercise safely and enjoyably through their pregnancies. In fact, the daughters of some of her first pupils have now also taken her classes!

Jane initiated Pregnancy Exercise classes at Crown Street Hospital in 1979, and since then has been first point of referral for many Sydney obstetricians whose patients are suffering from the musculoskeletal problems so common in pregnancy.

Since 1999 Jane has been teaching her increasingly popular classes at The Royal Hospital for Women, Randwick. She herself is the proud mother of Rachel and Talia.

POWERING
THROUGH
PREGNANCY

Keeping strong and supple for the most
important nine months of your life

JANE SIMONS

ALLEN&UNWIN

First published in Australia by Allen & Unwin in 2003

Allen & Unwin
83 Alexander Street
Crows Nest NSW 2065
Australia
Phone: (61 2) 8425 0100
Fax: (61 2) 9906 2218
Email: info@allenandunwin.com
Web: www.allenandunwin.com

National Library of Australia
Cataloguing-in-Publication entry:

Simons, Jane.
Powering through pregnancy: keeping strong and supple
   for the most important nine months of your life.

ISBN 1 74114 126 5.

1. Prenatal care. 2. Exercise for women.
3. Pregnancy. I. Title.

618.24

Model: Cara-Lee Poswell, now the proud mother of Aiden Gillis. Well done, Cara-Lee!
Illustrations: Ian Faulkner
Photography: Dave Bredeson
Internal design by Tabitha King
Set in 11/15 pt Rotis Serif by Midland Typesetters, Maryborough, Victoria
Printed by Griffin Press, South Australia

10 9 8 7 6 5 4 3 2 1

CONTENTS

PREFACE
WHY I WROTE THIS BOOK

Over the past 20 years or so there has been a radical change in attitudes to physical fitness in pregnancy. We have, thankfully, moved on from the time when women were told that the discomforts of pregnancy should be dismissed as part and parcel of the process of becoming a mother. In extreme cases, women suffering severe pelvic pain were often confined to wheelchairs or their beds. Now we know that there are specific exercises you can do, not only to remedy such problems, but also to prevent them occurring in the first place.

Attitudes to exercise vary, and pregnant women can participate safely in most forms of physical activity. Needless to say, however, there are the obvious exceptions and the bottom line must always be to use your common sense. One of my favourite images is of an acrobat from a well-known circus troupe who was still working as part of her team four weeks before the birth of her child! Not a course of action I would ever advocate, I hasten to add, but it is an interesting example of an elite athlete operating at the extreme end of the fitness spectrum, completely undeterred by her pregnancy. While most of us are far from being elite athletes, this does not affect my belief that, with common sense, most pregnant women can aim for and achieve their optimal level of fitness and wellbeing right up to the day they go into labour.

Over the years I have spent as a support-person/physiotherapist in labour wards I have also seen many changes in our approach to labour. It is no longer considered radical to kneel on top of the labour table — now women are encouraged and supported to give birth in the position that best suits *them*, not their obstetrician or midwife. We have also changed our attitude towards exercise during pregnancy. Having exercised with hundreds of pregnant women over the past 20 years, I am convinced, now more than ever, that it is never too late to address the issue of physical strength and flexibility. Obviously, the less fit you are the more careful you need to be and the more catch-up work you need to do, but nothing is impossible. I am constantly heartened by the words of new recruits to my exercise classes, who tell me that having been unsure of what exercise they could and couldn't do in pregnancy, they now feel lighter, more flexible and full of energy.

This is why I have written this book.

1
INTRODUCTION

This is such wonderful news. Your pregnancy test is positive and you are about to embark on the most exciting journey of your life. Congratulations! As the prospect of motherhood begins to sink in, you undoubtedly have a checklist of questions needing answers. Near the top of the list is probably the question of how you, as the mother-to-be, are going to maintain your physical wellbeing over the next few months. Being comfortable with the changes your pregnancy will bring is a significant part of physical and psychological wellness and exercises that specifically address these changes will keep you flexible, strong and feeling good about yourself.

As part of a normal pregnancy you must expect certain aches and pains as your body adapts to accommodate your growing baby. Keeping yourself fit and incorporating a regular exercise program into your daily routine will make an enormous difference in how you cope with these changes. Before commencing any exercise program, however, you do need to be aware of certain dos and don'ts which are covered in this chapter. In Chapter 2 we look at these aches and pains in more detail and how exercise can reduce any discomfort that they are causing you. You will learn to work with your changing body to make movement and exercise more comfortable – and enjoyable!

For many women, pregnancy is a magical experience filled with exhilaration, excitement and boundless joy. Buoyed by all this emotion, the majority of women in my classes report little difficulty dealing with the radical, and rapid, transformation taking place in their bodies. Others, however, are not as fortunate but, in my opinion, good levels of stamina, strength and energy make all the difference, as evidenced by the wonderfully healthy women I see in my exercise classes. I am convinced that being physically fit is essential to how you feel both within and about yourself, and how you will cope with your new role of motherhood. I hope that this book will help you achieve the 'personal best' that is possible for any woman at any stage in her childbearing life.

With hindsight, most women agree that motherhood is the hardest, yet most gratifying job they ever take on. It is the hardest in that it is both physically and emotionally draining. But the great news is that you can upgrade your strength and flexibility to ease the physical toll. Never be despondent about 'not being fit' and never be intimidated by those around you who appear fitter and able to exercise more efficiently than you. Today is the first day of the rest of your life and yes, you can make a difference. This sounds like a blatant sales pitch, but I have absolutely no doubt that the sooner in your pregnancy you start exercising, the easier it will be and the more benefit you will gain – especially if you continue exercising up to the day your baby is born.

I am often asked 'How soon after the birth can I start exercising again?' or 'How soon will I have my figure back?'. Both answers will depend on your pre-pregnancy attitude to physical wellbeing. Those who have enjoyed a regular exercise program before giving birth and who are committed to exercising after their baby arrives can be back to their pre-baby shape once the baby is six months old. In fact, in my experience, they are often thinner. Nonetheless, there are always the exceptions, with some women able to walk out of hospital in their jeans and others who take months, even years, to get back in shape. If you are one of the latter don't despair, for there is much that you can do and many people are prepared to help you achieve the body of your dreams. What matters most is that muscles stretched by pregnancy regain their former tone. It just takes a commitment from you.

That being said, while we all want to look our best, *please* remember that the childbearing year is the most physically taxing time of your life, especially in the early days after giving birth, so be kind to yourself. Don't beat yourself up about gaining weight — it is an expected part of pregnancy. The purpose of the exercises in this book is not to keep your weight down, but to boost your energy and strengthen the postural muscles you need to cope with the sheer physical load of pregnancy and new motherhood. Relax into this new phase of your life and accept that you will become a little rounder as your body lays down a few fat cells for emergency stores — never underestimate Mother Nature because she is never wrong. After your baby has arrived, a program of remedial exercise will soon have you looking good and feeling strong, ready to enjoy your new role.

It stands to reason that stamina and energy are boosted by regular exercise, but keeping fit has a secondary benefit in that it produces endorphins. These naturally occurring hormones help us feel good about ourselves, not only by increasing our stamina and energy but also by regulating mood swings. Most mothers-to-be are familiar with the emotional 'roller-coaster', but a program of regular exercise and keeping fit will temper these swings.

WHY DO YOU NEED TO BE STRONG IN PREGNANCY?

In my practice as a physiotherapist working primarily in obstetrics, I see pregnant women with a range of musculoskeletal problems (see page 74). It is interesting to me that a high percentage of these women fall into the category of non-exercisers. For a variety of reasons they have either given up exercise or have not done any specific strengthening or stretching exercises during their pregnancy and this has left them vulnerable to the normal complications of pregnancy. Once these women commence an exercise program designed to strengthen and stretch their muscles, however, their symptoms significantly reduce and they have a greater degree of independency and self-sufficiency. This helps them to deal with the normal, but sometimes overwhelming, changes that are taking place in their bodies.

Perhaps a good starting point is to give yourself a metaphorical 'pink slip' for physical fitness. (For those who don't drive, a pink slip is the checklist of a car's condition, which every car has to pass before it can be registered. This may seem an odd analogy, but many people treat their car better than they do their own body!) How did you do? Be as honest as you can, because this will give you a better idea of the amount of work you need to do. For some, this won't be much, but others will have a lot to do. No matter what the outcome, seize this opportunity to make some lifestyle changes that will, in the long term, give you that wonderful feeling of physical fitness and a healthy, toned and supple body. The stronger you are, the better able you will be to deal with the demands of the childbearing year. Your pregnancy hormones loosen your pelvic joints and weaken your pelvic floor muscles and, as a result, your abdominal muscles are subjected to an incredible amount of strain. Once your baby is born, sleep deprivation and continuous lifting and bending combine to leave you at greater risk of muscle fatigue and strain. With the right information and knowledge, however, and the appropriate strengthening programs both before and after birth, you will be fit, strong and able to enjoy the exciting journey ahead.

One of the most important byproducts of exercising during your pregnancy is the good residual level of fitness you will have after your baby is born, just when your time for yourself is at a premium. The fitness you achieve and maintain through your pregnancy will last for a good few weeks after you give birth, so take full advantage of being able to choose when and where you want to exercise and begin your exercise program now!

WHY DO YOU NEED TO BE FLEXIBLE IN PREGNANCY?

During your pregnancy you will hear a lot about hormonal softening and abdominal weakening, but very little about flexibility. Although they know that specific areas are softening up in preparation for giving birth, many of the women in my classes still complain that they feel a need to 'loosen up'. This stiffness can be explained by a number of reasons:

- your baby's presence under your diaphragm produces a characteristic protective posture, or lifting of the ribcage, which can lead to stiff and sore shoulders and upper back. To begin with, this 'guarding' may be more psychological than physical, but as your baby grows and your uterus takes up more space under your ribs and then your lungs, this guarding posture becomes unavoidable. Your normal range of movement becomes more limited and your upper back stiffens, which causes that rolling or 'waddling' gait so characteristic of pregnancy;
- it is natural to compensate for the change in the size, shape and weight of your breasts either by lifting your shoulders too much or too little, adding to your upper back stiffness;
- spontaneous movement can cause unpredictable aches, pains and twinges, so it's natural that your movements become more premeditated or stiffer;
- and last, but not least, many women are apprehensive about movement of any kind, not only because they don't know what is or isn't safe, but also because they want to cushion their growing baby from any possible harm.

All of the above are legitimate and understandable reasons for this stiffness, but specific stretching exercises and knowledge can alleviate the problems.

THE MUSCULOSKELETAL NEEDS OF PREGNANCY

Throughout the book, I will be talking about the musculoskeletal needs of pregnant women. These are:

- a strong back;
- a flexible back;

- core control (abdominal muscles that effectively support your growing baby and help you maintain good spinal posture);
- strong legs;
- upper body strength; and
- a responsive pelvic floor.

The exercises in this book are designed to address all of the above but, before commencing your exercise program, you must be aware of the specific aches and pains that occur as part of a normal pregnancy. While you may not be experiencing any of them right now, they could present at any time and need to be managed appropriately. I strongly recommend that you read through Chapter 3 before you begin your exercise program.

THIRTY-SOMETHING FIRST-TIME MUMS

Many women are choosing to have their babies later in life and most of them have already realised the value of keeping fit as they juggle the demands of their hectic schedules. Long work hours can mean extended periods of sitting at a desk and keeping fit can be vital in reversing any resulting back strain.

Maternity leave, both during your pregnancy and after your baby is born, is meant to ease the transition to motherhood and you should use this time to come to terms with the fact that you need to slow your normal pace and take more care of your physical wellbeing. This may mean that you have to rationalise not only your career demands but also your daily chores. Women are no longer 'married to the house' and domestic chores can be shared, ditched or ignored, if you can! It's not easy to relinquish control of your household, especially since you have absolutely no control over what your new baby will do from one minute to the next, but try to accept gracefully any offers of help that will let you grab a precious half-hour for yourself.

Another factor that causes many women to give up exercising is the (false) idea that exercising uses up precious energy. Actually, the reverse is true. Any amount of exercise, no matter how little or low-key, energises and refreshes. You may feel tired immediately after a class, but I promise that you will feel more energised the next day. I also believe that 10 or 20 minutes of exercise refresh more than an extra hour of sleep, but you will never know unless you give it a try.

HORMONES, MOOD SWINGS AND EXERCISE

Bombarded by a barrage of emotions, you can't help but reel under the onslaught of your hormones, both during your pregnancy and especially after giving birth. Unsurprisingly, this affects your energy levels and it is normal to feel low at times, and disinterested in exercise. There are many ways to deal with the 'baby blues', but poor fitness levels can leave you feeling even more downbeat. Gentle exercise is the least invasive and most natural way of regulating your mood swings, so if you find yourself feeling a little gloomy go for a walk around the block and let the fresh air pick you up. You can take baby with you, in a pouch or in her buggy, as she will enjoy an outing too.

THE IMPORTANCE OF MODERATION AND REST

When your baby arrives you will find yourself on a physical and emotional roller-coaster, with energy levels that fluctuate from one extreme to the other. For the first few weeks you are cushioned by the 'happy hormones' of new motherhood, but then the cumulative effects of sleep deprivation kick in. Baby sleeps through the night, then she doesn't, then she fools you by doing it again, but this time you are lying wide awake, worrying that there is something wrong with her! And so it goes. Welcome to the world of sleepless nights. Get as much rest as possible and start practising that balancing act that women are renowned for. Try to fit in a little exercise when you can and you will soon feel, and see, the benefits.

EXERCISE AND THE THREE TRIMESTERS

THE FIRST TRIMESTER

This is a time when pregnancies can be vulnerable and some women are advised to take it easy, but others can exercise as normal. The bottom line is that you must consult with your doctor to find out whether or not exercise is appropriate for you. The first trimester is often associated with morning sickness and many women feel too nauseous to do anything, let alone exercise. Many women also feel very tired through the early weeks of their pregnancy — if this is you then it's natural that you don't feel like exercising. Don't force yourself to do too much. Hopefully you will soon start to feel more like your old self and then you can start an exercise program.

THE SECOND TRIMESTER

This is often the time in your pregnancy when you will feel at your best and able to exercise as much as you want. While the normal aches and pains of pregnancy often present at this time, they should not stand in your way if you take the remedial measures covered in Chapter 2. If you do this, you should be able to establish an exercise program that you can continue (and enjoy!) through to your due date.

THE THIRD TRIMESTER

At this stage in your pregnancy you may feel like you are back at the beginning again — tired and nauseous, with heartburn or indigestion thrown in for good measure. Or you may feel absolutely wonderful! Common sense dictates that as you get heavier you will need more rest but it is still possible to exercise regularly. Most of the women in my exercise classes can carry on with the program up to the day their baby is born.

WHERE DO YOU START?

Before commencing any exercise program, read the following guidelines and check with your doctor that it is appropriate for you to be exercising. There are several major contraindications to exercising while you are pregnant. If any of the following conditions apply to you, you must get the 'all clear' from your doctor before starting any exercise program. Some of these contraindications are temporary and, if your doctor approves, you can begin exercising once the condition has either responded to the appropriate medical advice or intervention, or resolved itself.

CONTRAINDICATIONS TO EXERCISING IN PREGNANCY

- A history of miscarriage.
- A history of premature labour.
- Cervical incompetence which has been treated with a stitch.
- Vaginal bleeding or loss of fluid.
- High blood pressure.
- Any sudden or unexplained pains in your abdomen.
- Your baby isn't moving.
- Fever.
- Suspected or confirmed deep vein thrombosis in your legs.

GUIDELINES FOR EXERCISE DURING PREGNANCY

- Confirm with your obstetrician that there are no abnormalities or underlying complications in your pregnancy that could prevent you from exercising.
- If you have not exercised for a while begin gently and increase your level of activity gradually.
- Drink at least the recommended 1.5 litres of water a day and always have a water bottle with you during the warmer months of the year. You should always drink water before and after exercising.

- Stick to the list of 'Golden Rules' in Chapter 2 (page 18).
- Build up to exercising at least three times a week for about 45 minutes to an hour each time.
- Use your common sense. If at any time you have any questions about your exercise program, check with your doctor, physiotherapist or midwife.
- Use your pregnancy as an opportunity to establish long-term healthy lifestyle changes.

NEVER

- Exercise to the point where you become overheated or exhausted.
- Exercise in hot conditions.
- Follow up any exercise session by sitting in a sauna or spa as this can cause your body temperature to rise to dangerous levels.
- Water-ski, as accidents can result in water penetrating your vagina.
- Hold your breath as you exercise, as this can cause extreme fluctuations in your blood pressure. In fact, holding your breath should be avoided not only during your pregnancy but at any time of exertion.
- Use exercise as a method of weight control during your pregnancy.

Guided by the above recommendations, you can exercise safely up to the day your baby is born, so let's get started!

2
PREGNANT
AND FIT

Throughout this book I will talk about a wide variety of muscles and how to exercise them, but there is one specific group that forms the basis of many of the exercises – the abdominal muscles, the building blocks of postural support. These muscles are so important that I have covered them in some detail, and included precise anatomical descriptions. Please take the time to familiarise yourself with this additional information before commencing the exercise program, as these muscles are not only pivotal to postural support; they are also the mainstay of core stabilisation.

CORE STABILISATION

Core stabilisation is a term that you will come across frequently throughout this book. Your 'core' is your spine and 'stabilisation' is provided by its enveloping and overlapping muscles which provide a strong foundation of support. In turn, this strong foundation enables our limbs to work more efficiently.

Let's picture our arms and legs as a system of simple levers. As with all levers, their base of support is critical to how well they work. A common example of leverage in action is the crane on the building site with its long, moveable arm anchored to its mechanism on the ground. The more effective the bracing or support for these moveable limbs, the more efficiency and safety there is in their use.

While many of us treat our bodies like a mechanical device, a fundamental difference between the crane and the human body, other than the obvious, is that we need to be as concerned about the condition or safety of our anchoring mechanism as we are about the effectiveness of our limbs; this anchoring site is, of course, our spine. Most of us are either oblivious to this fact or choose to ignore it. I am not alone in believing that this disregard for our core muscles as we go about our day-to-day activities is the root of all back pain.

As I have already mentioned, core stabilisation not only protects the spine but is essential for the efficient use of our limbs. You will feel this for yourself when you try the following exercises. Bracing these core muscles makes certain exercises much easier to do. Effective stabilisation can be learned in an exercise class and applied to specific exercises but it is much more important to put it to practical and daily use. It is essential to your back's wellbeing and must become an automatic action.

Core stability is a team effort, a result of the synchronised bracing of many different muscles, tightening in all directions. These muscles are the deep abdominal and back muscles together with the pelvic floor; ironically, the very ones most affected in pregnancy – the abdominal muscles have to stretch to accommodate your growing baby and the pelvic floor is softened by your pregnancy hormones in anticipation of labour.

It should go without saying that throughout the childbearing year these muscles need to be as toned and responsive as you can get them, and in my experience this is best achieved by exercise. The women in my classes who exercise regularly are very successful in upgrading their strength and tone.

The abdominal muscles are also called the abdominal 'wall', although they could just as easily be renamed the abdominal 'corset', as in fact they wrap around the waist like a thick band or belt attached on either side to the spine. The abdominal muscles are the most 'switched off' muscles in the body, as evidenced by the number of men and women walking around with 'pot-bellies'. If the abdominal muscles aren't firing, there is little support for the abdominal contents, which means that the back muscles or spine itself have to take up the strain. It is this overload that causes back pain. But there is a simple remedy. Brace your abdominal and pelvic floor muscles to reinstate the support and your back pain disappears almost instantaneously.

The bad news is that this supportive bracing needs to be in place 24 hours a day, seven days a week, and the moment we turn it off the pain returns. The good news is that managing back pain at any time in our lives is very much within our control — we simply have to strengthen our core muscles and learn how to brace them effectively. With practice, this bracing will become automatic.

Bracing the abdominal and pelvic floor muscles is naturally much harder in pregnancy. As your baby grows, your abdominal muscles are pressed forwards and your pelvic floor has to support the extra weight of your baby, while it is being softened by your hormones. But if we stop working with these muscles, they will be further weakened and stretched. Both muscle groups are well able to contribute as part of the 'stabilising team' as your baby grows, remaining strong and reactive to the day your baby arrives.

It's understandable to be apprehensive that bracing your muscles will harm the baby. I remember feeling exactly this, feeling so protective of this precious bump. Your baby is a passive little being, but she will let you know if any activity you are doing is not to her liking. In fact, she will wriggle and kick and let you know in no uncertain terms!

As an added bonus (or side effect, call it what you will), I am beginning to suspect that women who exercise these core muscles to the day their baby is born have less abdominal separation of the rectus muscle (see page 15) after the birth. Stretching the abdominal muscles (see the exercises on pages 24–30) and keeping them well-toned and firing throughout the nine months of your pregnancy, will ensure that they return to this pre-stretched state in a matter of weeks after you give birth. Obviously a post-natal exercise program is part of this recovery process, but if you were committed to exercising before the birth, you will be just as committed afterwards.

FUNCTIONS OF A STRONG ABDOMINAL WALL

Strong abdominal muscles are:

- the mainstay for good posture;
- the mainstay for spinal support;
- a key component of core stabilisation;
- the diaphragm's partners in performing expulsive movements such as in childbirth; and
- able to contain or hold the abdominal contents in their designated positions, while gently yielding to internal pressure from the growing baby.

The abdominal muscles look like this.

ANATOMY OF THE ABDOMINAL WALL

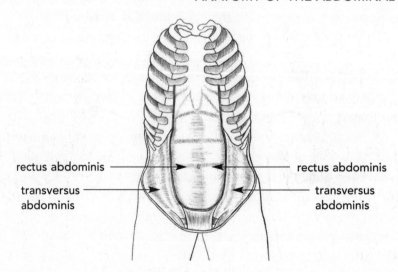

rectus abdominis   rectus abdominis

transversus abdominis   transversus abdominis

TRANSVERSUS ABDOMINIS (TA)

This is the corset muscle, the deepest layer of the abdominal wall. It is a significant contributor to the stability of the lower back. From its attachment point at the back to the spine, it wraps from one side of the spine through to the belly button in the front to join up with the corresponding transversus muscle on the other side of the waist. Bracing this muscle with a gentle, low-grade but sustained contraction should and can be done for long periods of time, in fact all day. The majority of back pain sufferers aren't very aware of this muscle, yet once they learn to switch it on and keep it on, their pain usually abates.

THE RECTUS ABDOMINIS

The rectus abdominis or 'six pack' muscle demarcates the area where separation occurs in pregnancy. As your baby grows, the abdominal wall is stretched to the point where it can stretch no longer and then the process of separation or

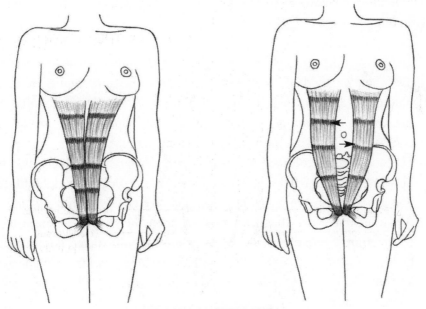

ABDOMINAL SEPARATION

yielding begins. What this means is that a gap develops between the parallel muscles running down from the centre of the rib cage to the centre of the pelvis. This muscle separation can be felt both in the latter stages of pregnancy and after the birth but the gap will close with the passage of time, provided you have been diligent about exercising both before and after the birth.

PELVIC FLOOR

Pregnancy is a time for many lifestyle changes, one of which is becoming aware of your pelvic floor. Becoming super-tuned to pelvic floor control will stand you in good stead for the after-effects of birth. You can begin these contractions now, as you read, as this is the one exercise that can be done any time, any place, anywhere. If, however, your muscles are particularly weak, you will be much more effective in strengthening them if you put time aside specifically for these exercises.

Begin by identifying the two types of contractions — fast-acting and slow-acting.

- The fast-acting contractions shut the external sphincter. It's the action we use when we suddenly feel an urge to go to the toilet and there is none around. To exercise these muscles feel a short flick or contraction around the ureter or opening to the bladder. Do about 20 or so of these contractions at a time in a rapid repetitive action.
- The slow-acting contractions exercise the deeper supportive pelvic floor muscles and are felt high up into the vagina. Begin by tightening the muscles around the vagina, anus and ureter, the three openings in the perineum. Now you have some idea of the overall strength of this contraction. Try to divide this contraction into four stages, contracting bit by bit, four times until you feel you have tightened or drawn in as deeply as you can. Hold for as long as you can then release down in a similar four-step fashion.

Feeling the hold at the top requires a great deal of concentration. Repeat these four-step contractions until you reach your fatigue level. Fatigue level is the point where the muscle can no longer respond to your voluntary command and the muscle needs to rest before commencing exercise again. You may find your fatigue level is five repetitions, you may find it is 20. Before recommencing exercise, you will need to rest for at least 20 minutes.

COMBINING THE FAST- AND SLOW-ACTING CONTRACTIONS

Repeat this four-step contraction and hold as deeply as you can. Add ten of the fast-acting contractions, then slowly release all your muscles. Repeat the double contraction until you reach your fatigue level. Repeat this sequence throughout the day and aim to do anything up to 100 contractions or ten bunches of ten per day.

Now that you have an awareness of how to do a full pelvic floor contraction and know the difference between the fast- and slow-acting contractions, you can do these sequences little and often throughout the day, every day, for the rest of your life.

HOW DO YOU KNOW IF THE PELVIC FLOOR IS WEAK?

In pregnancy the signs of a weak pelvic floor are:

* a leakage of urine when coughing, sneezing, straining to lift a child, running and even laughing;
* a feeling of heaviness in the perineum; and
* an inability to stop the flow after urinating.

The benefits of maintaining or restoring your pelvic floor strength are:

* maintaining bladder and, in some instances, bowel control;

- easing the feeling of engorgement in the perineum especially towards the end of pregnancy;
- easing the pain of haemorrhoids;
- easing the pain of vulval varicosities (varicose veins) in the perineum;
- easing a painful coccyx;
- easing the pain of pubic symphysis; and
- correcting vaginal flatus (air popping in and out of the vagina).

COMMONSENSE GUIDELINES—A FEW GOLDEN RULES

As you begin your exercise program, *please* follow these recommendations:

- **When stretching, exercise in your comfort zone.** This means only moving to either the point of limitation of movement or to the point of pain. Repeating the same movement over and over again usually increases your range of movement. Be gentle on yourself and adhere to the 'comfort zone' rule as overzealous stretching can cause micro-trauma leading to further tightness. Repeating each exercise in the pain-free zone for a minimum of five repetitions will usually ease any discomfort, including most back or pelvic pain. If pain increases, however, stop the exercise immediately and try an alternative soothing movement. Seek medical advice from an experienced obstetric exercise therapist or your doctor if you are concerned.
- **Sustain each stretching hold for at least two in-and-out breaths.** This will elongate, or remodel, tight tissue.
- **Breathing freely at all times is of paramount importance.** You should make your breath work for you and breathing freely increases your flexibility and range of movement. It also helps you to relax. Many women find yoga and Pilates both helpful and enjoyable forms of exercise in pregnancy. One of the strongest features of both these exercise disciplines is the emphasis they place on correct breathing. You can use

the outward breath to help you complete the more active phase of each movement. Never, ever, hold your breath for any reason.

- **Use your fatigue level as a guideline as to how many repetitions of an exercise you should do.** You will be able to complete a set number of repeats of an exercise before your performance drops off, when you are unable to maintain the elements of precision and accuracy. This is your fatigue level. Stop and rest when you reach this point, then continue if you wish with the same exercise or move on to another.

- **Sustaining or holding each strengthening exercise will 'fire up' or activate muscle fibres.** Weak muscles are ignored muscles. Strengthen your muscles slowly and deliberately, bombarding the muscle fibres with nerve impulses. This will switch them on and make them come alive.

- **Back pain is often transient and can disappear after gentle repetition of a movement.** You may find that the first movement hurts but subsequent movements become more and more comfortable, until you are pain-free. This is not to say that the pain will not return, but exercise will similarly alleviate any further episodes of pain.

- **Familiarise yourself with the '10-point' posture check'** on page 20 and be sure to implement this for any exercises in standing or sitting.

- **Check your base of support.** When you are in the standing position you should be in the 'knees-over-feet' position (see page 20). Your feet should be hip width apart, parallel to each other with the knees positioned directly above the first and second toe. Check the posture of the foot muscles as well. Keep your weight distributed over the outsides of your feet, not your arches. This not only preserves your arches, but also forces you to engage all the muscles in your feet, legs and hips. This means that your knees and ankles will remain stable and you can work your leg as a whole — from the tips of your toes right to the top of your hip! Once you are in the correct position, you will find your hip and pelvic muscles working strongly to give maximum support to the pelvis.

10-POINT POSTURE CHECK

- Stand with your feet hip-width apart and your knees slightly bent.
- Let your arms hang loose beside your hips.
- Get a sense of how you carry your body weight, starting from your feet and working through your pelvis to the top of your head.
- Check your foot posture.
- Your body weight should be distributed evenly over the outsides of your feet, your heels and your toes.
- Check that your knees are positioned directly over your second toe.
- You should feel your buttock muscles engage to support you in this position.
- Tuck your chin in and lengthen the back of your neck
- Check that your lumbar spine is in neutral. Your lower back should curve gently inward and be braced by your tummy and pelvic floor muscles.
- Be sure to keep breathing freely throughout.

Now you can begin to correct your spinal posture. Starting from the base of your spine, pull yourself up to your full height. You will feel each of your vertebrae decompressing, from your coccyx up to the base of your skull. Your back, tummy and pelvic floor muscles are now working in harmony to lengthen and elongate the whole of your spinal column.

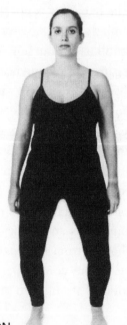

KNEES-OVER-FEET POSITION

THE EXERCISES

EXERCISES

Belly button brace
lying on back

Belly button brace
on hands and knees

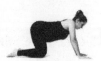

Belly button brace in sitting

Belly dancing in
standing

Belly dancing
leaning on a wall

Belly dancing on
hands and knees

Belly dancing
supporting chin

Butterfly

Draping in standing

Spinal twist in
standing

Rotations in side
lying

Push-ups

Clams

Side scissors

Double straight
leg raises

Bridging

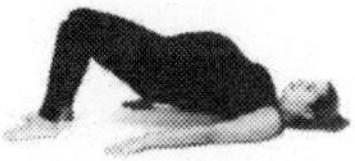

Chin draping

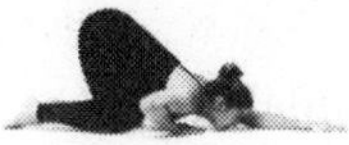

Chin draping
against a wall

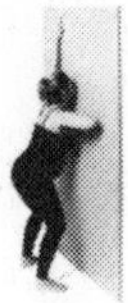

Draping

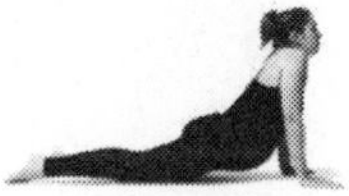

Squatting

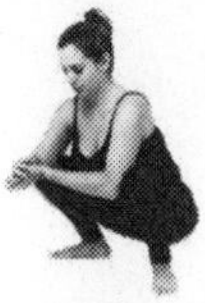

Leg swinging

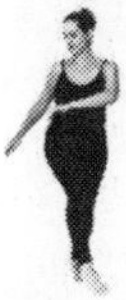

Forward tip

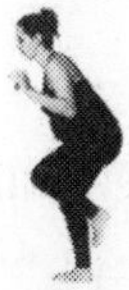

Belly dancing
on a ball

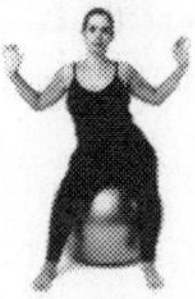

Side stretch

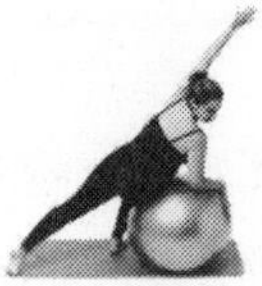

Rollaway

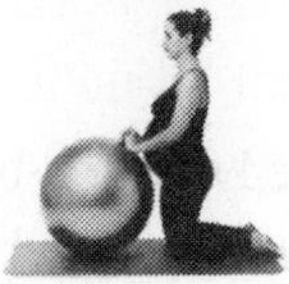

Side-to-side roll

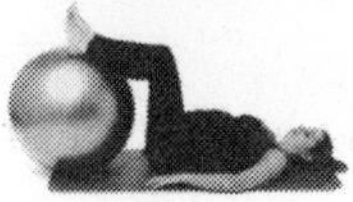

Bridging

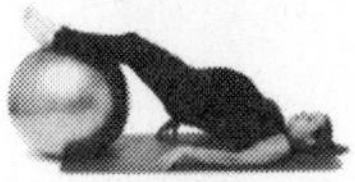

Pelvic lift

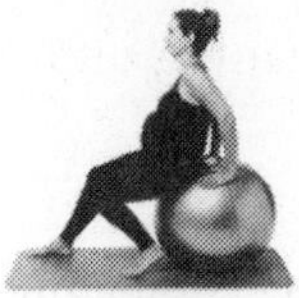

Posture challenge

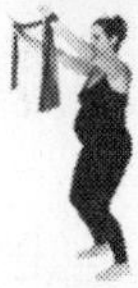

Asymmetrical
posture challenge

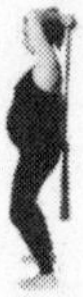

Double posture
challenge with
side bend

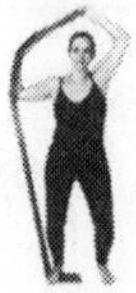

BELLY BUTTON BRACE

This exercises the deepest of the group of abdominal muscles, those representing nature's internal corset. Contracting these muscles narrows the waistline; the primary internal support for your spine. Training these muscles can be done in many positions, including lying on your back, in the hands-and-knees position and, most importantly, in sitting.

Useful cues to help you learn how to do these exercises would be to try to narrow your waistline imagining you are trying to zip up tight jeans.

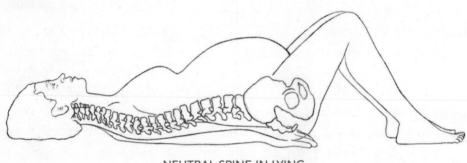

NEUTRAL SPINE IN LYING

BELLY BUTTON BRACE LYING ON YOUR BACK

- With your knees bent up, correct your lower back posture to ensure it is in neutral. Neutral spine is the natural spine alignment that places least stress on the spine. To find your neutral spine you must engage your abdominal muscles. Exercising in neutral spine protects the spine from injury while forcing the abdominal muscles to work properly. As you are lying down, your lower back should be relaxed. If there is a space between your lower back and the mat, bend your knees up to your chest and gently circle your legs, holding your knees with your hands. This will relax your lower back when you return your legs to their original

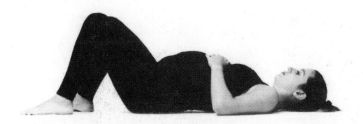

position. Gently lengthen your neck so that your head is moving away from your shoulders, but do not tilt the top of your head into your mat, or tuck your neck and chin. You should now feel comfortable and supported – you are in neutral spine.

- From this position, start by breathing in towards your belly feeling your belly button ease outwards then, as you breathe out, tighten your pelvic floor and brace around your belly button, drawing it downwards over your baby and towards the spine. You should feel the sides of your waist narrowing. This is a gentle tuck requiring concentration, not power. When you are on the right track you will feel a pressure-like sensation at the sides of the waist and, most importantly, no movement of the ribs or pelvis. Your tail bone should remain anchored to the floor.
- Contracting these muscles squeezes the belly button closed. A visualisation that might be helpful is to imagine there is a diamond in your belly button and you are trying to grip it in there.
- Repeat the motion until you have a clear idea of how it feels, then add a 5-second hold at the end of the outward breath. Your lower back should remain in neutral at all times and don't forget your pelvic floor contraction.
- Now try it in the hands-and-knees position.

BELLY BUTTON BRACE IN THE HANDS-AND-KNEES POSITION

- Your hands should be directly under your shoulders, your knees under your hips and your spine in neutral. Don't let your back sag downwards.

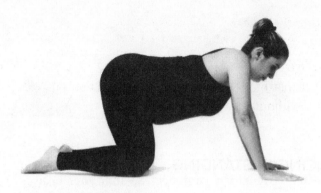

Breathe in and let your belly sag down towards the floor while maintaining your spine in neutral.

• As you breathe out, squeeze your tummy muscles up against your baby to press it and your belly button back up towards the spine. Tuck with your pelvic floor and then squeeze for 5 to 10 seconds. This is a subtle contraction that requires concentration and thought. The learning process may be frustrating, but once you get the hang of it, it is something you will have no difficulty in implementing 24/7. The 5- to 10-second hold will help you get the feel of this contraction and the gentle build-up of power it brings.

• Initially many women feel a need to hold their breath, but once you have the knack of the belly button brace, you will easily be able to brace independently of your breathing. Bracing independently of your breathing is an integral part of many of the following exercises.

BELLY BUTTON BRACE IN SITTING

Perhaps the most important time to brace is during prolonged periods of sitting. Brace in exactly the same way as above, maintaining your neutral spine and feeling your waist narrowing.

BENEFITS

This is the primary abdominal contraction used in posture correction and spinal support. It partners the pelvic floor contraction and many believe one cannot contract without the other.

BELLY DANCING IN STANDING

This is a classic exercise, useful both during your pregnancy and after. Belly dancing is the gyration or twisting motion of the pelvis enjoyed as an art form and exercise by many cultures throughout the ages. It requires controlled pelvic movement and is a very effective exercise to highlight abdominal muscle control and soothe back pain. It is used extensively in labour to ease the pain of contractions.

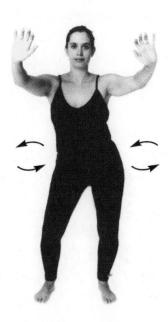

- To begin, prepare by checking you are in the knees-over-feet position.
- Carry out the '10-point posture check' on page 20.
- Hold your arms out to the side both for balance and to activate the muscles around the thoracic spine.
- Slowly rotate your pelvis in as wide a circle as you can manage, using your buttock, abdominal, pelvic floor and lower back muscles. You should aim for a smooth, controlled action, and should feel the movement in both your lower and mid-back.
- Reverse the direction to rotate the other way.

BELLY DANCING LEANING ON A WALL

Place your elbows at shoulder height in front of you on the wall. Lean towards the wall to support your upper body while you belly dance in exactly the same way as above.

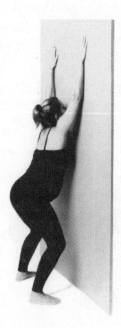

Your core stabilisers or internal corset – the back, buttock, thigh and pelvic floor muscles – will brace your belly button to your baby, your baby to your spine.

BENEFITS

This exercise strengthens your stomach muscles. It is good for mobilising stiff backs as well as relieving the pain of contractions.

BELLY DANCING ON HANDS AND KNEES

This version of belly dancing is more a journey of discovery which you can use to identify painful spots in the lower back or pelvis. Of course, you may not find painful spots and simply enjoy the wide range of movement in your comfort zone, where you are completely pain-free. If, however, you do discover trouble spots, the idea is to move in ever-increasing circles and enjoy the soothing effect of movement. This movement is very effective in labour to reduce the pain of contractions, especially if you are feeling a lot of back pain.

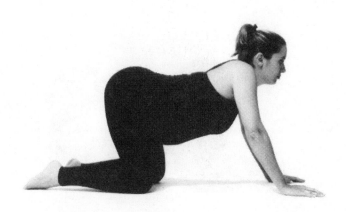

- Start on your hands and knees, with your hips directly above your knees and your shoulders above your hands. Notice the surge of relief when you first get into this position as you eliminate gravity's drag.
- Begin rolling your pelvis in a random fashion searching out those painful spots and trying to nudge out tightness.
- Of course, you may not have any painful spots. If so, this motion will maintain your spine's range of movement.
- Feel the bracing effect from your tummy, buttock and pelvic floor muscles as they propel the pelvis and support the baby and your spine.

BELLY DANCING SUPPORTING YOUR CHIN

In this position you can get in touch with any discomfort or stiffness in the upper back between your shoulder blades. This movement feels wonderful if your upper back is aching.

- By supporting your head in your hands you anchor the top of the spine, letting the rest of your back drape naturally.
- This draping action is enhanced by the free circling of the pelvis in an up/down or round and round action easing out any tight spots you may discover as you circle.

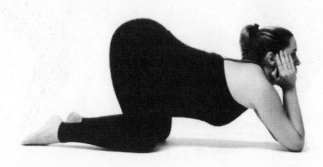

- You will probably feel this stretch most at the level of your bra strap. To stretch different areas of your upper back you will need to vary the position of your elbows by walking them either forwards, backwards, closer to each other or outwards.
- This rolling action is also a toning exercise for the tummy and buttock muscles.

BUTTERFLY

This exercise is a form of pelvic tilting done in the standing position, a rhythmical flow of the whole of your spine from flexion to extension.

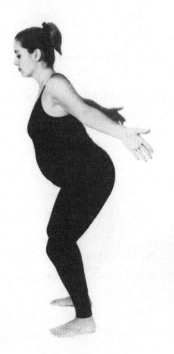 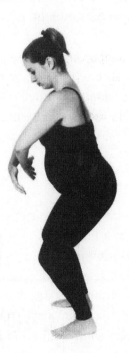

Throughout both phases of this movement your tummy and buttock muscles will be working strongly to control both the curl and the arch of your back, while you use an arm movement that resembles the sweep of butterfly wings.

- Start with your knees bent in the knees-over-feet position.
- Check your body weight is forward over your feet, your lower back arched to neutral.
- Beginning with the curl, breathe out as you tuck your pelvis with a tummy, buttock and pelvic floor contraction, wrapping your arms gracefully around your chest like the wings of a butterfly to engage the upper abdominal muscles.
- Breathe in, release the curl and begin to extend; opening out your arms and lengthening your whole back, lifting the rib cage and pushing your pelvis back with a strong contraction of all the back muscles.
- Curl, breathe out and add the pelvic floor crunch to the flexion phase.
- Extend, breathe in as you open up and arch.

BENEFITS

This exercise strengthens your tummy, back and buttock muscles, while improving the flexibility of your spine.

DRAPING IN STANDING—IN THE KNEES-OVER-FEET POSITION

This exercise is most effective to relieve your aching back after you have been sitting for a long time.

During the curling or tummy-crunching phase, feel the releasing of the lower back muscles, an ideal movement to do 'on the run'. This requires strong leg and buttock work to stabilise the pelvis.

While you may find the first movement uncomfortable or even experience sharp pains in the sacro-iliac, mid-back or lower lumbar area,

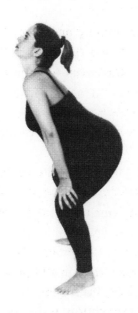
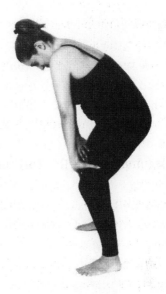

don't give up but repeat the movement **within your comfort zone**. The more repetitions you do, the sooner the discomfort will ease and disappear. If you are still experiencing pain after 10–20 repetitions, consult your doctor or physiotherapist.

- Begin in the knees-over-feet position, gripping your knees with your hands.
- Brace your buttock and hip muscles to ensure your knees do not drift towards each other. This also engages the supportive muscles that protect the pelvis.
- Sink your body weight through your locked elbows towards your knees and feel the 'drape' or extension of your torso and spine.
- Reverse this position by flexing or rounding up the spine. As you flex, gently shift your body weight to your heels, flexing the lower back with an abdominal and pelvic floor contraction and buttock squeeze.
- Repeat this flexion/extension movement 5–10 times to feel its mobilising effect on the whole spine.

BENEFITS

This exercise improves the mobility or range of movement of your spine, and is a good flexion stretch for tired back muscles. It also strengthens your stomach muscles, wrists and arms.

SPINAL TWIST IN STANDING

This exercise targets your mid-back or thoracic spine, the area most affected by prolonged periods sitting in front of the computer or long sessions of feeding your newborn.

Adding the twist to the previous exercise brings in the movement of rotation, the primary movement of the mid-back. Throughout the exercise, your body weight should be distributed evenly through both feet and knees. Check that your knees do not drift inwards towards each other as you twist

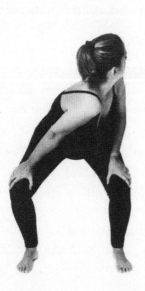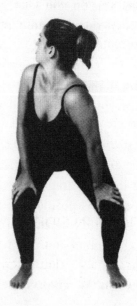

from side to side. Maintaining this correct position will ensure that rotation occurs in the spine, not in the ankles.

* Begin in the knees-over-feet position, as for the previous exercise, with your body weight spread evenly through both arms.
* Keeping the left elbow straight, allow your right elbow to bend and slowly rotate to the right to look up and back over your shoulder. This produces the mid-back rotation. As your left shoulder dips down you can feel the stretch between the shoulder blades. (With all these elements in place this exercise feels like a complete wringing out of the spine, a wonderful feeling of twist.)
* Reverse the direction to rotate to your left, bending the left elbow and straightening out the right, to look over the left shoulder.
* Breathe freely throughout the rotation, holding the stretch for at least one outward breath. This should last for at least five seconds for you to get the full benefit of the stretch.

With practice you will find you automatically brace the muscles around the pelvis to stabilise it during the movement, but initially you should concentrate on the sensation of twist in the middle back.

BENEFITS

This exercise is a passive rotation of the whole spine, which will maintain and extend your flexibility. It is also a gentle lengthener for your tummy muscles and will strengthen your wrists.

ROTATIONS IN SIDE LYING

This is a class favourite, a total unravelling of the whole spine. Do not despair if at first you are unable to reach the floor with your elbow – the first movement

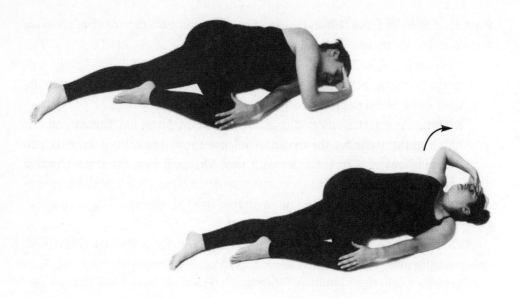

always feels stiff. Repeated movement increases range — some women find they get to touch the floor after a few repetitions, others take weeks, some never manage it. Some of us are stiffer by nature so simply rotate to 'your end range', working in your comfort zone at all times. Never lift your head off the floor, simply roll it over throughout the movement from one side to the other.

- As shown above, lie on your left side, holding your right knee down with your left hand and placing the fingers of your right hand over your forehead.
- Keeping your head in contact with the ground at all times, slowly roll your head and elbow over to the opposite side and try to touch the floor with your right elbow.
- Stay with this stretch for at least the length of a full outward breath, then return to the starting position and repeat the movement slowly, stretching deliberately, breathing freely and holding the movement at end range for the duration of a couple of in and out breaths or at least ten seconds.

- Rotate to the point where you feel either discomfort or limitation of movement in any part of your spine or torso. You will find that this discomfort abates as you repeat the movement. If you are in the last trimester your baby will be pressing your abdominal wall forwards and you may feel a strong stretch, perhaps even discomfort in your upper abdominal muscles and ribs on the side you are lying on. Should you feel this tightness during the exercise, release the hold on your knee as you rotate allowing it to roll over with you. This will ease the discomfort on the side you are lying on, but you will find that this discomfort diminishes in intensity after a few repetitions.
- Repeat the movement at least 10 times to one side.
- Before rolling to the opposite side, protect yourself from round ligament or abdominal pain by preparing for the roll as described on pages 75–8 'rolling over'.
- Repeat the process with the opposite arm and leg combination. You will be surprised at how quickly your spine loosens up. Pay attention to any different sensations between the two sides of your body – you may find that one side is a little more flexible than the other.

Each time you begin this stretch you may be a little stiff, uncomfortable or even experience sharp pains in the sacro-iliac, mid-back or lower lumbar area. Do not give up, simply repeat the movement in your comfort zone and any discomfort will abate. If you do this stretch every day, you will maintain (your individual) full-range rotation for life.

BENEFITS

This is an excellent stretch for your torso muscles. It also increases and maintains spinal rotation.

PUSH-UPS

Whenever I demonstrate this modified push-up there are howls of protest from the class as it looks harder than it really is. The point of this exercise is to strengthen the arms while challenging the stabilising action around your baby and lower back. As your pregnancy progresses, you will find that turning from side to side becomes harder, and this exercise prepares your arms and upper body to help you. You may find it difficult at first, but it will get easier as your arm muscles get stronger.

- Prepare by bracing your deep abdominal muscles, pelvic floor and deep back muscles to restore neutral spine.

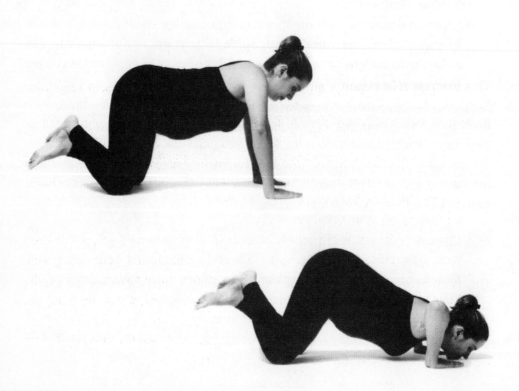

- Bend your elbows and try to dip your chin to touch the floor in front of your fingers. The closer your hands are to your knees the easier it is to dip, the further away they are, the stronger the bracing action required.
- Dip your chin only to the point where you can still maintain the brace of your abdominal and back muscles.
- As soon as you feel your back and tummy sagging, stop, and return to the start position.
- Repeat up to your fatigue level, which may be only 5 or 6 repetitions.

BENEFITS

This exercise strengthens your shoulders and wrists, while challenging your tummy and back stabilisers; all of which helps with turning from side to side and rolling over in bed.

CLAMS

This exercise relies upon a strong corset of transversus muscles to keep your body steady throughout the movement. You must make absolutely sure that you are in the correct starting position and follow all of the steps below.

- Lie on your side with your elbows bent and pointing upwards above your head, your fingers pointing down the back of your neck. Your hips and knees should be bent at an angle of about 60 degrees. Your head should be resting on your underneath arm.
- Brace with the whole of the torso. This means belly button brace, pelvic floor tuck, tight buttocks, lumbar spine braced in neutral and your upper back muscles braced with your shoulder blades drawn down towards your pelvis.
- Your top hip should be positioned directly above the hip you are lying on. Try to maintain this alignment throughout.
- Your underneath knee should be pressing so hard into the floor that your underneath hip is almost lifted off the floor.

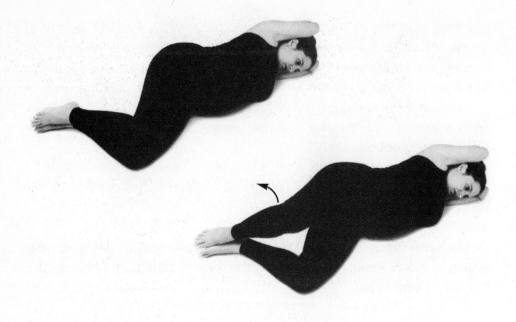

- Your elbow and forearm on the same side should also be pressing hard into the floor, to the point where your ribs feel they may be lifting off the floor.
- If you are correctly braced, you will find you are tilted fractionally forwards and this is your starting point.
- Open and close the top thigh, making sure that you keep your heels together throughout the movement. You should be able to feel the transversus muscle working, especially as you close the knee downwards.
- Consciously engage the muscles in your back and draw your shoulder blades downwards, away from your ears so that your pelvis remains motionless throughout and you are not rolling back or forward.
- You should feel your hip and thigh muscles working hard. These muscles are essential for stabilising your pelvis as the bones and ligaments shift and soften in preparation for labour.
- Turn carefully through your arms (as described on page 77 'rolling from side to side') to repeat the movement on the other side.

This exercise strengthens your corset muscles, as well as giving your hips, thighs and buttocks a good work-out.

SIDE SCISSORS

This exercise targets similar muscle groups to 'clams', but according to the members of my class, it's harder!

- Lying on your side, your head resting on your extended arm, brace your belly muscles and draw up your pelvic floor, making sure your spine remains in neutral throughout. Draw your shoulder blades down, away from your ears, and make sure that you are not sagging into the mat through your waist. You should be able to fit your fingers into the gap between your waist and the mat.
- Place your upper hand on the floor in front of your breast bone to help you balance.
- Breathe in to prepare. As you breathe out, raise your upper leg, with your foot flexed or pointed, to just above hip height keeping it raised throughout the exercise.
- Raise your bottom leg to meet the top one.
- Slowly lower the bottom leg, making sure not to touch the floor, then raise again, repeating this movement 10 times before you turn through your arms to the other side.

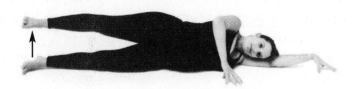

- As you raise and lower your lower leg, feel your corset muscles switching on and off. Concentrate on maintaining a neutral spine throughout this exercise and be sure not to roll from side to side as you lift your legs.

BENEFITS

This is a strong exercise for the transversus abdominis, buttock, hip and thigh muscles.

DOUBLE STRAIGHT LEG RAISES

- In the same starting position as for the previous two exercises, check that your top hip is positioned directly above the one you are lying on. For an added challenge, you can raise your upper arm straight up in the air.

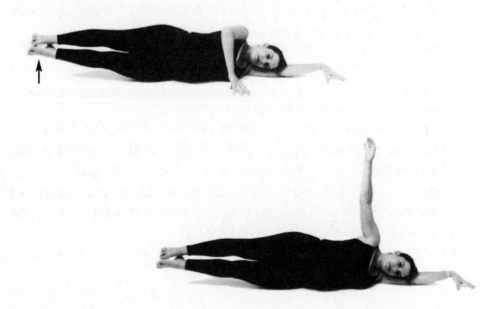

- Check your neutral spine, both lumbar and cervical, bracing with your core postural muscles (pelvic floor, tummy and back muscles). As you breathe out, lift both legs sideways, remaining steady on your side as you lift. Breathe in as you return to the start position.
- You should feel your core stabilisers working hard, and your muscles around your pelvis bracing as you lift. Repeat this movement 10 times.
- Repeat on the other side, remembering to brace before you turn over by lifting yourself through your arms.

BRIDGING

This is a basic back exercise which you can use to monitor levels of pelvic or back pain. If you feel any discomfort as you prepare for this exercise, powering up (increasing the depth of the contraction) your buttock, pelvic floor and tummy muscles as you lift will instantaneously reduce the level of discomfort. If you're still not convinced, try a few more repetitions and you will notice a difference. This exercise is a good example of the importance of making sure you are in the correct starting position.

- To start, lie on your back with your spine in neutral. Your knees should be bent up and your feet parallel, hip width apart and tucked in close to your bottom.
- Bring your shoulder blades together, breath in, then release the breath and brace your stomach muscles in preparation. Then, squeezing your buttocks, begin to lift, first rolling your pelvis off the floor, then your spine until your hips, knees and shoulders are aligned. Your tummy and back muscles will work together with your buttock muscles to control the movement of your pelvis.
- At the top of the lift make sure that your body weight is being taken by your shoulders, not the back of your head.
- Hold the lift for a full breath, then as you breathe out, slowly reverse this

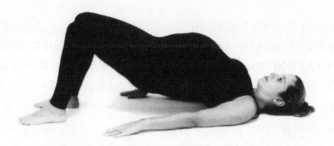

rolling action, lowering your shoulder blades first then uncurling the spine, vertebra by vertebra, until the pelvis has rolled down to the floor. Your tail bone should be the last part of you to reach the floor.

- Once you have the rhythm of this movement you will feel equal bracing from your lower back, upper back and shoulder blade muscles, as well as your tummy, pelvic floor and buttocks.
- Make sure that your tummy muscles brace throughout and repeat the whole process 10 times.

EASIER VERSION

For those of you who are a bit out of condition or who feel a twinge or two as you lift, place your hands under your buttocks and use them to help you raise and lower your pelvis. As the muscles around your pelvis get stronger, you will find you no longer need your hands and can complete the raising and lowering movement with them by your side on the floor.

HARDER VERSION

You can take this exercise to the stage where you raise and lower your pelvis repeatedly, at no time touching the floor beneath you. Raise your pelvis to end range, or as high as you can go, then lower only until your spine touches the floor, your pelvis remaining just off the floor. Your tummy muscles are braced around your baby throughout. Repeat this movement to your fatigue level, which at first may be only 6 repetitions, but ultimately you should have no trouble completing as many as 20. As with all the exercises in this book always increase your repetitions gradually. This exercise can also be done on the ball, and the method is described on page 63.

BENEFITS

This is a good strengthener for your abdominal, buttock, thigh and back muscles.

CHIN DRAPING

The thoracic spine (between the shoulder blades) is a notorious trouble spot in women, probably because our breasts cause us to be too conscious of posturing or bracing this region of the spine. This exercise is a great opportunity to stretch and lengthen the muscles both in front and behind the rib cage.

- Start in the hands-and-knees position, with your hands positioned beneath your breasts and knees hip width apart.
- Stretch one hand in front of you, sinking your body weight forwards and extending your arm to the point where your body weight is spread equally through your chin and the extending arm.
- Feel the stretch of the pectoral muscles, together with the suspension of your spine, which targets the mid-back to produce a feeling of pressure between the shoulder blades. The trick to this exercise is to share your body weight between your hands, chin and knees, varying the slide of the moving hand to target the stretch in your mid-back. The lower your pelvis is towards your heels, the more effective the stretch is.
- If you do not feel the stretch between your shoulder blades, check the position of your supporting hand, which should be directly under your

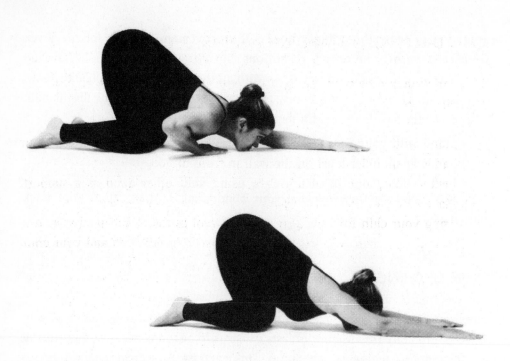

breasts. If you still don't feel the stretch try shifting more weight on to your chin until you can feel the pressure between your shoulder blades.

- To return to the starting position, take most of your weight through your supporting hand under your breasts, while simultaneously drawing back your extended arm.
- Repeat on the opposite side.
- Finish with a double stretch, stretching both hands forward. To return to the starting position, sink down onto your elbows then walk them back to the start. Double stretches will further mobilise or add pressure to the spine at the level between the shoulder blades. Repeat the double stretch several times.

CHIN DRAPING IN STANDING AGAINST A WALL

This variation can be successfully done in standing, so it's more practical for busy lifestyles.

- Stand with your feet hip width apart and knees slightly bent. Place your hands at shoulder level on the wall in front of you.
- Begin sliding one hand upwards, using your other hand as a support. Make sure you share your body weight between both hands.
- Bring your chin forward to rest on the wall as the upper hand stretches, so that you share your body weight between both hands and your chin.

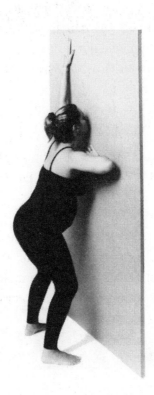

You may need to adjust the positions of your hands and chin to target the stretch to specific areas of tightness.

This is a wonderful passive stretch for your thoracic spine, pectoral muscles and tummy muscles.

DRAPING

Many women are apprehensive about this exercise, but the key points to remember are to limit the stretch to the duration of one outward breath and stretch only in your comfort zone. As you practise this exercise it will become more comfortable and you will feel a general sense of stretch throughout the upper abdominal wall, groin and lower back. Many women find that this exercise becomes a firm favourite as they near their due date.

- Starting in the hands-and-knees position, prepare by taking most of your upper body weight through your arms and shoulders.

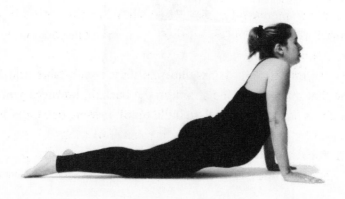

- Then for the duration of one outward breath, drape your tummy and as much body weight as feels comfortable, hanging from your shoulders and limiting the stretch according to your level of comfort.
- Don't drape too far or you may find yourself stranded and unable to return to the starting position.
- This is a powerful stretch through the abdominal wall to the groin and lower back, so hang only for the length of the outward breath.
- After a few repetitions you can reverse the movement by sitting back on your heels with knees wide apart or going into the squat position.

BENEFITS

This is a strong stretch for the groin and lower back, and a gentle lengthener for abdominal muscles. Stretch within your comfort zone and you will find that it will ease the burning sensation around the ribs common in later pregnancy.

SQUATTING

Many cultures use this position as a way of life but, if you plan to use it regularly, bear the following points in mind. Squatting requires you to be flexible through the joints of your knees, hips, ankles, Achilles tendons and calf muscles. Most importantly, you must have good circulation in your legs. If your circulation is poor, and especially if you have varicose veins, squatting is not recommended.

Not everyone is able to assume this very comfortable and functional position, one that puts little or no strain on the back. If, however, you are in the habit of using this position and feel no build up of pressure or congestion in your legs, use it to feel a wonderful stretch in the whole of the pelvic area.

Squatting is an excellent position for relieving the pain of pubic symphysis. You may initially feel a strong sense of stretch around the centre

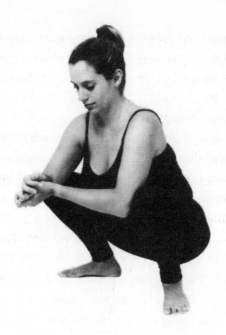

of the pubic area as you sink into the squat, but this is usually followed by a significant relief of pain. You may need to practise squatting daily, as the pain relief is only temporary.

Although squatting flexes the lumbar spine it is not as stressful as flexion in sitting where the spine is compacted. There are many things that can be done in this position, so if you are one of the lucky ones comfortable while squatting, make it a way of life while caring for young children. You can also try doing pelvic floor contractions while you are squatting. And if you have trouble squatting with your feet flat on the ground, squat on your toes.

- Start in the hands-and-knees position with your knees and feet as wide apart as is comfortable for you.
- Walk your hands back between your knees towards your heels to sink your weight through your pelvis.

- As you sink, relax your lower back completely and feel the stretch deep into the pubic symphysis and your lower back. You may feel 'clicks or crunches' in the lower back region as you do this movement. Provided that the movement brings relief, just ignore them.
- If you find the pressure on your legs too uncomfortable, walk your body weight forwards out of the squat, back into the hands-and-knees position.
- Repeat this several times until you feel more comfortable.
- Squatting is an acquired movement or position that may take weeks to feel comfortable. If the squatting position doesn't come naturally to you, be wary of pressure building up in your legs especially if you are retaining fluid in your legs and feet. In such cases squatting will feel most uncomfortable and it is advisable that you don't persist with this movement until after your baby is born.

BENEFITS

This strong stretch offers significant, if temporary, relief for both pubic symphysis and sacro-iliac pain. It is also a good lower back stretch.

LEG SWINGING

This is a lovely movement once you get the rhythm going, but it requires strength and balance. Poor balance is not caused by pregnancy, only made worse by it, so if your balance is poor now is the time to try to improve it using this exercise.

- Begin by holding your arms out to the opposite side for balance and tune in to the bracing action of all the muscles around the standing leg.
- Swing one leg across your body concentrating on your balance and feeling the bracing and stabilising activity in your lower abdomen as well as the standing leg.
- Keeping your eyes on the floor in front of you will help you maintain

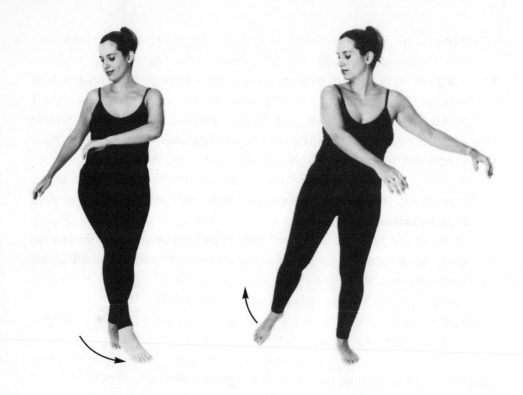

your balance. Once you feel secure with the leg swing, add an arm swing, moving your arms in the opposite direction to your leg.

• You will feel the bracing response of the transversus abdominis below your belly button and around your baby.

• You can vary the direction of the swing, from front to back and from side to side.

• Swap legs and swing the other leg.

BENEFITS

This movement strengthens your abdominal, thigh and back muscles. It also offers a gentle spinal rotation and challenge to your balance.

FORWARD TIP

This is a great movement to increase your pelvic stability, and teach you how to bend and lift safely. As a new mum, you will feel that you do nothing but bend and lift, so why not transform this unavoidable movement into a muscle trainer? Once you have all the elements of safe bending in place, each of these bends will not only protect, but strengthen.

- Throughout the movement keep your spine in neutral by bracing your back and abdominal muscles.
- Tip at the hip, contracting your buttocks as hard as you can. Using your arms for balance, tip to the point where you can grasp a small object (such as a toy!) off the floor with your right hand. Your hips act as a fulcrum and your right leg will come up behind.
- Return to the upright position, constantly bracing your buttocks, thighs, back and tummy muscles to stabilise your spine.

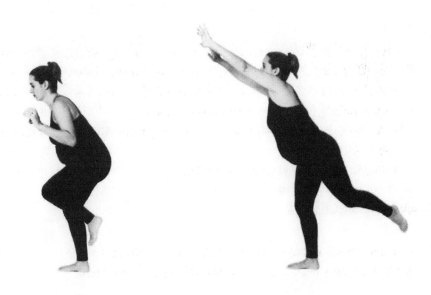

- You can add a degree of difficulty to this exercise by rocking up and down on the same leg. Repeat this several times and then switch to the other leg.

BENEFITS

This is an excellent back and thigh strengthener, and will protect your spine during lifting and bending. It's great for improving balance, for anyone of any age, so get your mum and grandma to join in!

BALL EXERCISES

It is a heap of fun to be part of a class full of pregnant women belly dancing on their balls. If you have never exercised on a ball you may need a little time to get used to the motion but in no time at all you will feel secure and comfortable, enjoying all the benefits they have to offer. The ball is an unstable base, which adds an extra challenge to the core stabilisation exercises. These exercises may prove to be hard work at first, but they get much easier with practice.

A ball is a great alternative to a chair, especially if you spend long hours in front of a computer. I would never have finished this book without mine. They are also very useful for easing pelvic or pubic symphysis pain, and can be used as part of your pain-management strategy for labour.

These balls are ready available in most sporting shops and some specialist furniture shops. They come in a range of sizes. The 65-centimetre ball suits most, but there are 55- and 75-centimetre balls available for shorter or taller women. Your ball is the right size for you if, as you sit on it, your knees are a centimetre or two below the level of your hips.

SITTING POSTURE ON A BALL

Correcting for neutral spine is as important when you are sitting on the ball as it is in any other upright or sitting position. It is as easy to slump on the ball as it is in any other sitting position and the instructions for good posture are fairly similar. The basic difference between sitting on a chair and sitting on a ball is that your support is not fixed, which requires you to be continually adjusting your postural muscles.

With your feet placed comfortably apart on the floor in front, check that they are bent slightly less than 90 degrees. You may find that it is more comfortable to let your heels rise off the floor so you are bearing your weight through your toes.

Check that both your lumbar and cervical spine are in neutral. As you sit, your body weight should be equally distributed through your feet, thighs and pelvis. Ideally, your coccyx should not touch the seating surface. Your core muscles (abdominal, pelvic and back muscles) are braced at all times to stabilise neutral spine.

The beauty of sitting on the ball is that it eliminates static loading of any one point of contact with the seating surface. In other words, there is an ever-changing load on all of the weight-bearing structures, and no one muscle has to be 'on call' all the time. Your body weight is, of course, absorbed by the ball and this is very kind to the softening pelvis in pregnancy. Those with pubic symphysis or sacro-iliac pain who have to sit for long periods will feel much more comfortable sitting on the ball.

GOOD POSTURE ON A BALL   BAD POSTURE ON A BALL

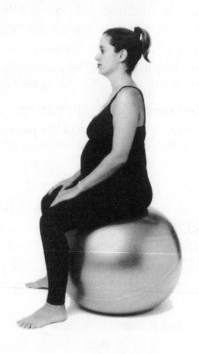
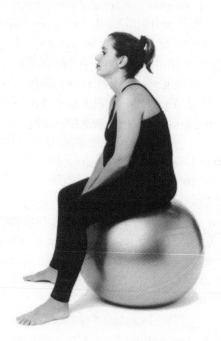

GUIDELINES FOR BALL EXERCISES

- Use your ball as an unstable base to challenge both balance and control. You must roll only to the point where you have the ball under the control of the muscles you are training.
- The more contact you have with the ball the easier the exercises will be – this is simple leverage. For example with 'legs on the ball' the hardest position is when only your heels are touching the ball; the easiest, with your thighs and calves on the ball.

- Before progressing try to increase the range or roll of the ball, making sure you are securely balanced and able to return to the start position. You will gradually increase your range with practice, but be confident with your current range before progressing to a larger movement.
- Sit slightly to the front of the ball and feel the base of support shared through your feet and pelvis.
- Hold your arms out as a tightrope walker does to help with balance.
- *Ensure AT ALL TIMES you have the '10-point posture check' in place.*

BELLY DANCING ON A BALL

If you have a ball at home use it as your seating option and you will find yourself doing the following exercises to relieve back discomfort.

- As you sit on the ball, implement the '10-point posture check' on page 20.

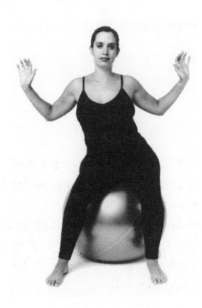

- Hold your arms out from your sides and draw your shoulder blades together until you feel muscle activity across your upper and lower back.
- Begin to roll the ball around in a circle. At first you will use your feet to roll the ball but, as you get used to the motion, use your abdominal, buttock and thigh muscles together to create the motion.
- Sweep the ball around in as large a circle as you can to feel the activity of the muscles enveloping your pelvis as well as movement in your lower and upper back.
- Reverse the direction of the roll and note how these muscles work differently.
- You may want to try this movement on your tip-toes, so that you are getting minimal support from your feet and maximum contribution from your pelvic muscles. This exercise is a wake-up call for all the postural muscles around your torso.

BENEFITS

This is a great exercise for dynamic abdominal bracing and postural awareness. It is also a good spinal mobiliser.

SIDE STRETCH

This looks a little scary if you have not done it before but feels very secure once you get the knack.

- As shown opposite, walk your feet to the left of the ball and lean your upper body through your right elbow.
- Grip the ball snugly with your right leg and stretch the left leg out to the side.
- Feel the stretch all down your left side as you reach over with the left hand.

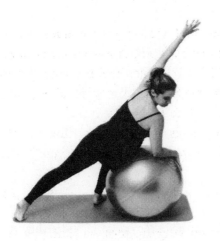 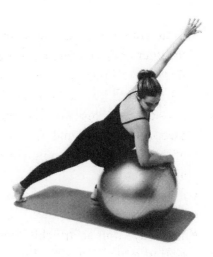

- Be sure to grip the ball with your open right hand and grip the floor with your left foot to stretch your left side as far as you can.
- Begin the rotation of your spine by turning your head to look down, then around and up. You will feel the full twist, or corkscrew, of your torso.
- Control the degree of stretch down one side of your torso by varying the height and position of your outstretched arm and by pointing through the toes of your outstretched left leg. In addition, you can thrust forward through the forearm you are leaning on.
- To return to the start position, sit back up to the centre of the ball by propelling yourself through your feet. Repeat the stretch on the opposite side, walking your legs to the right, leaning on the left forearm, thrusting through your right leg and right arm, turning to look back over the left shoulder.

BENEFITS

This is a great rotation stretch for the thoracic spine as well as a gentle motion to ease that burning feeling so commonly felt around the rib cage. It's also a good abdominal and groin stretch.

ROLLAWAY

This is a powerful challenge for your abdominal muscles and many new members of the class feel apprehensive about this exercise at first, as they are concerned it will place too much of a strain on the tummy. Once again, be guided by the comfort zone rule and always limit the stretch to the point where you maintain control of the roll.

- Start in the upright position with all your postural muscles in action and arms stiffened, with your elbows at right angles and hands clasped below the crest of the ball.
- Stabilise throughout your spine. This means draw down your shoulder blades, feel the upper and lower abdominal muscles tighten and brace your lower back in neutral.
- Now pivot on your knees, pressing your arms down hard into the ball to control the ball as it rolls forwards, keeping the spine in neutral.
- Feel the build up of power in your shoulders, upper abdominals and lower back and ensure your pelvic floor remains tight as the ball rolls out.
- Concentrate on being in control. Don't leave yourself stranded and unable to return comfortably to the starting position. In other words, roll only a distance you can easily return from while feeling a continuous spinal brace.
- Remember to maintain neutral spine and spinal bracing throughout the roll. Sagging as you roll will feel most uncomfortable but, more importantly, indicates that you are not in control of the ball.

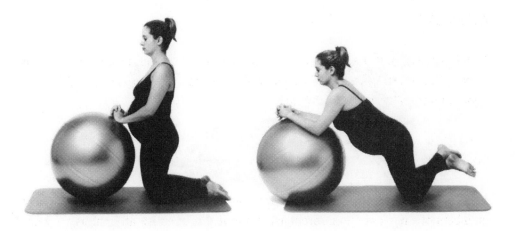

- Some are a little daunted by this exercise at first, so roll the ball forwards only a few centimetres and gauge your level of control. Increase the distance as your confidence and performance improve. The further away you roll the harder it is to maintain neutral spine.
- This exercise is best done by repeating small rolls in your comfort zone, slowly building up to the point where you can roll further by using the strength of your arms and shoulders.

BENEFITS

This is primarily a tummy, buttock and back stabilising exercise. It's also a good shoulder blade stabiliser and arm strengthener.

SIDE-TO-SIDE ROLL

Exercising on your back is perfectly safe as long as you are in motion all the time while doing a series of repetitions of a specific exercise. This exercise targets the transversus abdominis.

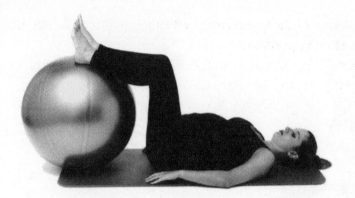

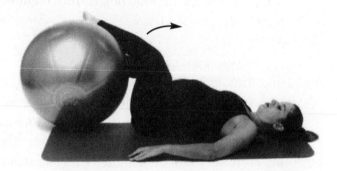

- Begin with your heels on the ball, your hips and knees at right angles, your legs lifted to a 90-degree angle.
- Make sure your lower back is in neutral and brace your lower abdominal muscles as well as your pelvic floor.
- With your arms positioned at a 45-degree angle on either side, feel the brace of your upper back and shoulder blades and maintain this brace throughout the roll.
- Maintaining neutral spine, breathe in and begin to roll the ball to the side to approximately 45 degrees, allowing your pelvis on the opposite side to roll up during the roll.

- Feel the bracing action of the transversus abdominis, and breathe out as you return to the starting position.
- Repeat to the other side being sure to stop at the start position before rolling to the other side. This gives you an opportunity to check that your spine is still in neutral and your muscles are braced before you roll to the other side.

HARDER VERSION

If you feel able to work harder do a series of small repetitions of the outward roll, rolling in and out at end range. This requires strong stabilisation, so only try this version if you are confident you can maintain neutral spine throughout.

BRIDGING ON A BALL

This is the same movement as bridging (see page 43), but this time with your feet on the ball. The difference now is that as you lift your pelvis the ball may begin to move. To steady the ball, you can use your arms on the floor by your side. As you become more proficient you can progress to finger-tip control. Ultimately, you will not need to use your arms and can point them up towards the ceiling as you lift.

- As you lie on your back with your feet on the ball, prepare with a belly button brace.
- Contract your buttock muscles, to roll your pelvis up off the floor until your knees and shoulders are in a straight line.
- Feel the muscles of your upper back joining in, to assist you with stabilising your torso.
- Practise lifting up and down and you will find it gets easier to remain steady on the ball. Use maximum support from your hands at first, until you feel safe and confident using only one or two fingers.

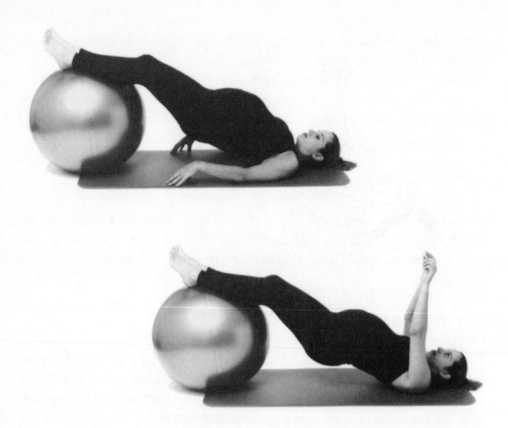

- Eventually you will be able to point your arms up towards the ceiling, using only your trunk muscles to stabilise. This last version is very difficult and should only be attempted once you can keep the ball steady during the lift.

BENEFITS

This is a core stabiliser that strengthens your back, buttocks and thighs.

PELVIC LIFT ON A BALL

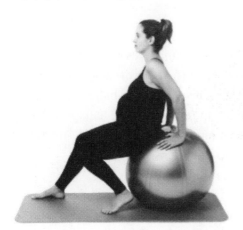

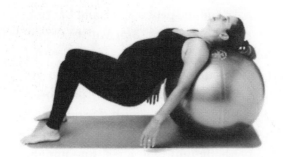

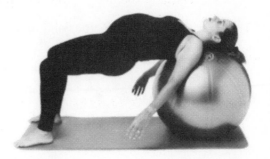

Getting into the correct position needs concentration. Take care that you do not fall sideways off the ball.

- To get into position, sit on the ball with your hands steadying you on either side of the ball and begin to walk your feet forwards away from the ball, simultaneously walking your hands back over the ball until you are in the position where your head and shoulders are on the ball, your knees at right angles and your hands trailing on the floor beside you, to steady you if necessary. You are now ready to begin.
- Start with the belly button brace to maintain neutral spine.
- Begin to lower then raise your pelvis without moving the ball.
- Once you are comfortable with this action, add the next step, which is to keep as much of your ribs as possible off the ball during the lowering phase, simply lowering and raising the pelvis only. This action calls for your transversus abdominis, pelvic floor and back muscles to stabilise as you lower and raise your pelvis. You will find that your buttocks and thighs are also working hard.
- Do not forget to add a pelvic floor contraction as you raise your pelvis.
- When you are ready to return to the start position, place your hands at hip level on the ball and begin to push down through your feet, walking them back towards the ball. At the same time push down with your arms to raise your upper body until you are sitting upright again.

BENEFITS

This exercise strengthens your abdominal, back, thigh and buttock muscles.

RESISTANCE BAND EXERCISES

The following exercises include the use of a latex or rubber resistance band. These can be purchased under different brand names at any good sporting goods outlet. The bands provide variable resistance to movement and come in different grades of strength. To suit your ability, you can choose a lighter or heavier grade, giving you more or less resistance. You can also vary the resistance of your band by either shortening or lengthening it between your hands. Obviously, the tighter the band the more resistance will be offered.

Secure the band by wrapping each end around your knuckles several times. Avoid gripping the ends with a tight fist as this can place strain on the wrist muscles.

POSTURE CHALLENGE

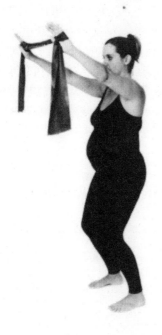
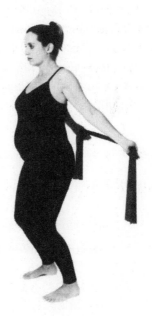

- Start in the knees-over-feet position and prepare by bracing your core muscles. Lift your pelvic floor, brace under your belly button and lift your baby towards your spine, all the time maintaining neutral spine. Feel your lower back muscles working to support this position.
- Maintain this bracing action throughout and challenge it by raising your arms out straight in front and stretching the band outwards. Lift your arms over your head then drop them behind your back. Throughout the movement make sure you draw your shoulder blades down towards your waist. This will add more tension on the band as your arms drop down behind your back.
- The response of your postural muscles as your arms travel up and over your head is critical to the effectiveness of this exercise. Ensure your neck remains in the neutral position (don't tilt or tuck your chin as your arms are raised and lowered). Ensure your lumbar spine is braced in neutral and you do not sag your baby forwards as you raise your arms.

Remember Effective postural support needs to be in place 24/7, and is achieved through sustained, low-grade muscle activity. This exercise trains you to tune in to those micro adjustments your postural muscles make in response to the movement of your arms and legs. For example, note how tempting it is to lift your ribs (as your tummy muscles switch off) as you lift your arms, or to protrude your tummy or chin when your arms drop behind your back. These are all common indicators of good posture disappearing.

ASYMMETRICAL POSTURE CHALLENGE

The technique and starting positions are the same as above, but this time one hand is directly above your head and the other pressed hard against your coccyx.

- Begin with the top elbow bent and pointing forwards, all your postural muscles firing.

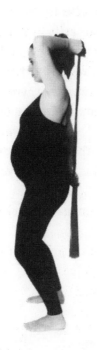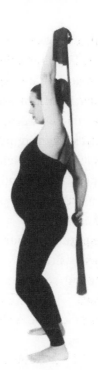

- As you breathe out, begin to straighten your elbow above your head. Feel the challenge to neutral spine, and to your postural muscles.
- As you breathe in, bend your elbow to return to the start position.
- Swap arms and repeat with the other arm bending and stretching. Swapping arms, repeat the movement 5 to 10 times for each arm.
- Check that the tension on the band is not too tight. You should feel comfortable resistance. You should not be struggling to straighten your arm above your head.

DOUBLE POSTURE CHALLENGE — SIDE BEND

- Secure the band as shown, with your heel anchoring it to the floor. Check that your hand pressed into the band is open, with your fingers pointing up towards the ceiling. As in the previous two exercises, you should be in the knees-over-feet position, with all your postural muscles firing, throughout the movement.
- Press your open hand into the band, feeling the resistance or stretch of the band. Begin to tip over to the side, bending from above your waist, to feel a sideways stretch on the way down. You should then feel the sideways muscular control of your postural muscles as you return to the start position.
- Breathe out as you bend sideways, breathe in as you return to the start position.

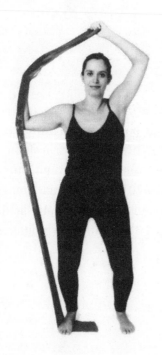
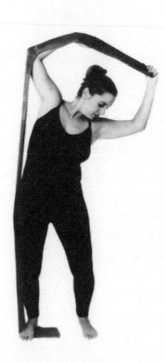

• Feel the postural challenge in both directions, from front to back as well as from side to side.

To feel the benefits of this exercise, you must maintain your postural brace throughout, and distribute your weight evenly through both your feet.

3

DEALING WITH SPECIFIC ACHES AND PAINS

Having read the guidelines and contraindications to exercise in Chapter 1, it is now time to familiarise yourself with the normal, pregnancy-related aches and pains. You may be one of the lucky ones who experiences none of the following symptoms, but let me reassure the majority who experience discomfort, however mild or infrequent, that this is very much part of a normal pregnancy and there is much that can be done to rectify it.

Pregnancy is a time when one can expect twinges of discomfort, when the aches and pains we look at in this chapter are considered normal. The degree of discomfort is variable and subjective and some mothers-to-be are unaware that these aches and pains are indeed attributable to pregnancy. The purpose of this chapter is to increase your awareness of what to expect and, should any of these conditions present, to equip you with pain-relieving self-management techniques. Most importantly, I want to stress that most discomforts are easily remedied and none will stop you exercising.

The following remedies and suggestions are designed to help you with your exercise program but obviously can apply not only to the exercises but to all movement in your daily activities. They will even help with basic manoeuvres such as rolling over in bed or simply getting up off the floor.

This is a list of the common aches and pains of pregnancy. The following pages will take you through each of these complaints and provide you with remedial or pain-relieving measures to help you manage and overcome these difficulties.

1. Aching lower back – pre-existing and unrelated to pregnancy
2. Sacro-iliac pain
3. Pubic symphysis pain
4. Aching between the shoulder blades
5. A burning feeling around the front of the rib cage
6. Coccyx pain
7. Round ligament pain
8. Swollen hands and feet

MANOEUVRING EASILY

Before we get down to the nitty gritty of dealing with specific aches and pains, we need to look at some simple manoeuvres as it is normal to feel a degree of discomfort while doing simple day-to-day activities. Rolling over in bed or getting in and out of the car can be tricky in pregnancy, but all you need to remember are a few basic tips to make these movements more efficient and comfortable.

BACK PAIN IN BED

Many women complain of back pain that seems to occur only while they are lying in bed. In my opinion, this pain is due to stiffness; this is confirmed by the fact that moving usually relieves the pain. The simple explanation is that we usually move around quite a bit while we are asleep. Pregnancy limits this spontaneous or subconscious movement and pregnant women find themselves lying in the one position for longer periods of time. If you wake with back pain, try squirming around in your bed, in a twisting, writhing motion. Begin gently, experimenting with movement in all directions and gradually increase your range of movement to nudge out the pain. Call this belly dancing, call it squirming, call it what you will but what you are doing is using movement to relieve stiffness-related pain.

PILLOW SUPPORT

Sleeping with a pregnant woman can become a bit fraught as she and her partner vie for the greater share of the mattress. Most pregnant women love to sleep with as many pillows as can possibly fit into the bed, for two simple reasons — support and comfort. So if you are having trouble sleeping because of restless legs or a sore back, place large continental pillows between your thighs and around your tummy, and cuddle up to an extra doona or even a beanbag, to get as much support as you can.

ROLLING OVER IN BED

Once you have decreased your level of discomfort or pain you will want to roll over to the other side. Prepare before you roll by bracing every muscle around both your lower and upper back or shoulder area. Bracing with the shoulder area while you roll propels the movement and reduces the effort required by the lower torso muscles. Bracing around the pelvis protects the loosening pelvis. To do this properly means squeezing with your buttocks, tummy, back muscles and thighs. This sounds like a lot to remember but it will become second nature after a period of training yourself each time you roll.

GETTING DOWN TO THE FLOOR

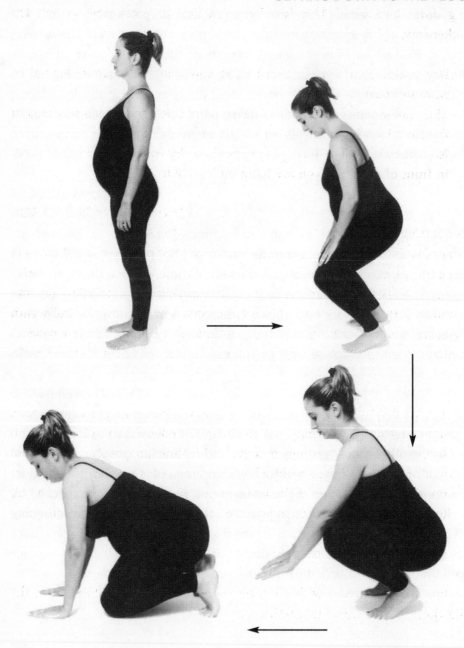

Getting down to the floor used to be a matter of bending in the middle then lying down backwards. This isn't very practical in pregnancy, so let's try another way.

* Begin with your feet hip width apart and your hands stretching out in front of you.
* Sink down onto your knees to the squat position then reach forwards to the floor to take your body weight through both hands.
* Now sit to one side. Lower your upper body by walking your hands along in front of you until you are lying on your side.

ROLLING FROM SIDE TO SIDE

Rolling from side to side is a movement you can not only use in bed but also during an exercise class or at a doctor's visit. As you will see, it is much easier if done facing downwards, but there are times when this is impractical and you need to do it the other way up. The first time you notice having difficulty with this movement will usually be at an obstetrician's visit where you have to negotiate that very narrow examination table. The following tips will make this easier.

* The first step is to transfer to the prone position, lowering to your side, not by using your tummy, but by using your shoulder girdle muscles to take the weight of your upper body. This requires support from both arms and bracing from the shoulder blade and upper back muscles.
* Continue with a brace of the lower back and tummy muscles, which will lock the pelvis and knees so you are able to roll as one, so reducing any possibility of strain.
* Reverse the order of this manoeuvre to get back up.

Use this bracing action with all turns where it is not possible to use the following more efficient alternative.

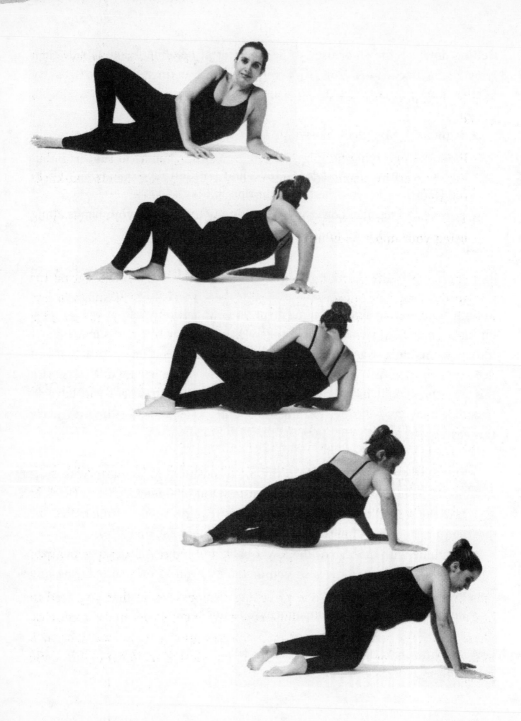

ROLLING FACE DOWNWARDS

This is the more efficient way to roll over and you can use it to roll over in bed.

- From the side-lying position, brace around your tummy to support it, but lift yourself by using your upper body to get to the hands-and-knees position.
- Then simply sit to the opposite side and lower yourself down once again, using your upper body muscles to do the lifting.

You can modify this position to roll over in bed. Here you do not lift all the way to the sitting position, but brace and swing your weight through in one movement. If this is too difficult revert to the previous roll using the leverage through your shoulder girdle.

GETTING UP OFF THE FLOOR

- Roll to the hands-and-knees position.
- Sink back into the squat position as on page 50.
- Simultaneously squeeze with your legs and buttocks, and place your hands on your knees. Lift your weight through your arms as they push down, to lift yourself up.

GETTING IN AND OUT OF A CHAIR OR BED

This process is similar to all the preceding manoeuvres, in that you need to brace the same muscles, but this time concentrating on your buttock muscles. These very large muscles are used to counteract gravity in all situations such as getting up off the floor or out of a chair, but most of us forget to turn these muscles on.

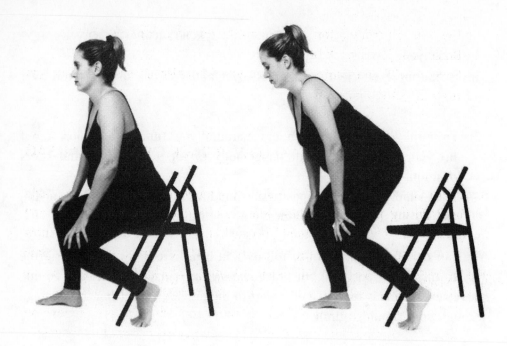

- Prepare before you move by bracing your buttock and leg muscles.
- Shift your weight to the front of the chair.
- Ensure your lower back is in neutral spine.
- Lift yourself, and notice how much easier and more comfortable this procedure is.

GETTING IN AND OUT OF A CAR

This will require the additional brace of 'keeping your legs together'.

- With knees together, sweep your legs sideways out of the door and place your feet on the ground.
- If necessary, use one hand under your thigh to assist with moving your legs.

- Use your other hand for leverage on the door frame of the car.
- Brace your lower back in neutral.
- Squeeze with your buttocks and use your shoulder muscles to elevate you from the sitting position.

ACHING LOWER BACK OR POSTURAL SAG

Back pain and back of the pelvis pain are separate conditions but are easily confused during pregnancy. Many women experience true pelvic pain and many experience back pain simply because they are stiff, and do not know how to move. Then there are the relatively few who experience true back pain arising from the spine. You will find it easier to differentiate these separate conditions as you read on.

Let's begin with some basic facts about spine care before we move on to detailed descriptions and remedies for pregnancy-related back problems.

Statistics tell us that at any given moment in time over 60 per cent of the population have 'back' pain, which includes all three areas of the spine, namely the lower back, thoracic or mid-back and the neck. A high percentage of back pain sufferers are mothers with young families, distracted from looking after themselves by the burden of responsibility and doing what mothers do best, putting themselves last. Neglect is a human condition that creeps upon us without our realising it, often becoming apparent only once we stop doing it. If this is you don't despair, for there is a lot you can do to remedy the problem – all you need is to find a little time to become more aware of your physical wellbeing.

When we are talking about the spine, we need to acknowledge how intricate and sophisticated it is – strong, supple and flexible, and able to conduct nerve impulses at the same time. It also has an early warning system – pain – that alerts us to the possibility of damage through mechanical strain. However, few of us recognise or appreciate these qualities, let alone work to preserve them. Not until there is a breakdown.

The system breaks down when we have gone too far, having ignored escalating discomfort or pain because we 'haven't got time'. It doesn't have to be a major event that causes back pain; it's more likely to be the cumulative effect of minor stresses repeated throughout the day that causes the damage.

We need to be constantly aware of our backs, so how do I get this message across? In desperation, I have chosen to appeal to vanity.

The spine's health is inextricably linked to the way it looks. Those with a healthy back are full of vitality and poise – they simply look great. From the physiotherapist's point of view a perfectly aligned spine reflects all the qualities of grace and elegance, hugely appealing physical attributes. So perhaps we should be appealing to our egos, to our body image, and then we might learn some lifelong good postural habits and spine care.

THE SAD TALE OF POSTURAL ABUSE

Pre-existing poor postural habits will usually get worse during pregnancy, but before we go into the reasons for this, we need to look at the basics of correct spinal alignment or good posture.

Most of us have no trouble admitting we do not pay enough attention to our posture. While we would not dream of failing to brush our teeth or wash our bodies daily, we deliberately ignore messages from our spines until either we are screaming out in pain or long-term damage has become irreversible.

The simple fact is that if any joint in the body is placed either under extreme or sustained mechanical strain, it will become either painful, damaged or both. Poor posture results in the skeletal system having to adopt a role it is not designed for, bearing our body weight without the support of our muscles. We simply slump, forcing the skeletal system to do work intended for strong, flexible muscles.

We compound this neglect with a lifestyle of poor lifting techniques. For example, does the sleep-deprived mother of two trying to load both the kids and the shopping into the car have the energy to think about or correct her posture? Probably not!

Another factor leading to back pain is poor muscle condition or, indeed, weakness, the back and tummy muscles being the main culprits. Weakness leads in turn to stiffness. It may seem paradoxical that a weak back can at the same time be a stiff one, but this is often the case. Stiff, inflexible spines can exacerbate pain as they are less forgiving to unguarded movements, such as trying to lift a cranky toddler who is desperate to be set down.

Many women face the added complication of the combination back. This is when hyper-mobility and stiffness co-exist. In other words, parts of the lower back are very mobile, but the thoracic spine is very stiff.

Trying to normalise these opposite conditions is a delicate process, in which we need to counteract one without making the other worse. It's tricky, but possible, and the key is to develop a keen awareness of what stiffness feels like, and what hyper-mobility feels like, and then be pro-active about remedying each.

Our spine has a genetically predetermined level of flexibility or range of movement and strain occurs when the spine is distorted or stretched beyond this point. Take, for example, lunging forward to snare a 'runaway' toddler. This movement can flex the spine beyond its full range and result in strains of the surrounding soft tissue. In this case, as with most others, if this particular mum has a flexible, strong spine she will be able to utilise a greater range of movement as she reaches forward, while her flexible, elastic muscles will respond automatically to guard her back and reduce the likelihood of injury.

Another very obvious example of overstepping range is with poor neck posture, where the postural muscles are 'abandoned' for the full slump posture illustrated on the following page. Here the neck joints are strained and this type of distortion often goes unnoticed for a number of years, pain manifesting only much later on.

This example shows the neck in a sustained, overstretched posture in which the joints are positioned far beyond their ideal or neutral position.

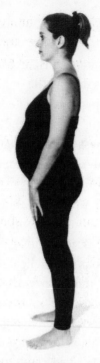
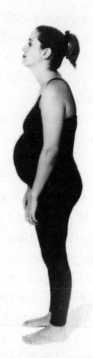

<table>
GOOD POSTURE | POOR POSTURE
</table>

GOOD POSTURE   POOR POSTURE

Such a posture cannot fail but produce neck, shoulder, arm pain or the lot.

Strong spines are also generally more resilient. A breast-feeding mum with a strong spine might be distracted and relaxed in an over-flexed position for extended periods of time, but she will not experience any back pain once she stops feeding, because of her on-going good postural habits.

WHY IS POOR POSTURE SO COMMON?

Many people seem to think good posture hurts, or that it requires lots of muscle strength. Of course it will be uncomfortable at first, if the muscles are not fit for the job! Expecting to have good posture when you have lazy, underused muscles is a little like putting a two-stroke engine into the body of a Ferrari. It just won't work! The solution, however, is simple, and is first to condition or strengthen your postural muscles and then practise good posture 24 hours a day, seven days a week.

POSTURE CORRECTION

Pregnancy results in a shift of your centre of gravity as your muscles brace in a way that is sometimes inappropriate and possibly can cause pain. Let's look first at what good posture feels like and then we can see how simple adjustments apply just as much during your pregnancy and will leave you more comfortable or even pain-free.

The essence of posture correction is to stretch tall, then actively maintain this correct alignment. Like any tall, vertical structure the spine needs good foundations in order to stay upright. If the foundations are not sound, there is the risk that the whole structure will topple. The spine's foundation comes from *core stability*, namely strong tummy, back and pelvic floor muscles. No muscle works in isolation, however, so strong thighs, buttocks and legs are also important. Good posture depends upon toned muscles throughout the body and can only be as good as the weakest link.

Good posture needs to become imprinted in our subconscious, an automatic action that we sense and activate all day, every day. Although pregnancy brings the extra challenge of compensating for the baby's weight out in front of you, the process of posture correction remains the same – some requiring only a little fine tuning, others needing to start from scratch. So let's check what it feels like.

- Standing with your feet hip width or comfortably apart, and your weight distributed evenly between both legs, stretch upwards slowly from the nape of your neck to reach your maximum height. (This may take at least ten seconds.)

- Feel the decompression from the base of your skull right down to your coccyx — the lengthening of the whole spine.
- Feel your spine realigning as the natural curves return to the neck, middle back and lower back.
- You will feel your deep tummy, back and neck muscles working to hold these curves.
- Recognise the correct position for your head. Your chin should be tucked, and you should be able to draw a straight line down through your ear lobes, shoulders and pelvis.
- Tune in to your centre of gravity, and feel your body weight distributed through the middle of each foot, rather than your heels or your toes.
- You should be breathing freely.
- Your arms and shoulders should be quite relaxed.

Try this in standing first, then in sitting. You will soon realise that it is much harder to have good posture in sitting.

CONTRAST TRAINING

As good posture is all of the above, challenge it with a contrast activity. Try correcting your posture as described above, feeling the contributions from all the supportive muscles, then reverse the movement. Slump and sink down. Straight away you will feel a compression throughout your whole body and notice that the natural curves of your spine have become distorted or exaggerated. Your muscles have failed to anchor the neutral alignment of the spinal column.

Tilting or slumping not only produces a feeling of compression but, worse than that, take a look in the mirror. How you have aged! And it's not only you. Take a look around you and notice the effects of poor posture. And this has nothing to do with a person's age, because many elderly people have wonderful posture, and just as many young people have shocking posture. Now do the opposite, stretch tall, activate those anti-gravity or postural muscles and take another peek in the mirror. See how the years disappear?

Good posture is an 'either/or' situation.
You either have good posture or you don't.
Either gravity wins or you win.
Don't let gravity win!

MEASURES TO RELIEVE PAIN FROM TIRED, SAGGY BACKS

In addition to the exercises in Chapter 2, the following may help to relieve pain.

- Lying on your back, bring your knees in to your tummy and gently clasp your hands over your shins. Feel the self-massage, as you roll your knees around in a circular pattern. A number of rotations should ease out any discomfort in your lower back. Breathe freely at all times.
- If you are still feeling sore then continue with this next exercise. Still lying on your back, squeeze your tummy muscles around your baby and tighten your bottom muscles hard. Press your lower back into the floor, lifting your coccyx slightly off the floor. This reverses postural strain and should be repeated little and often to eliminate pain.
- Try the same movement in standing. This is of course the basic pelvic tilt (see page 19), only this time in standing. It's also an effective pain-management technique in the hands-and-knees position. Do this in conjunction with postural correction as much as possible.

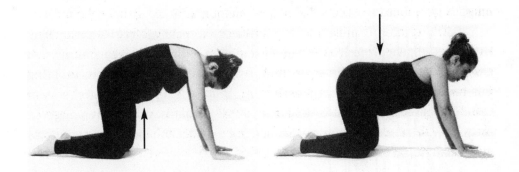

* Belly dancing in all positions relieves pain in your lower back. Belly dancing leaning on a ball is particularly effective.
* Kneel in front of your ball and hug the ball to your breasts.
* Turn your head to one side and rest your cheek on the ball.
* Move your hips in a slow, circular movement as in the earlier belly dancing movements on pages 27–30.

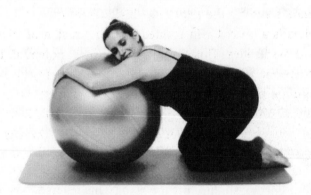

SACRO-ILIAC PAIN

This is the most common musculoskeletal discomfort experienced in pregnancy and often described as 'back pain' or 'sciatica'. It is, in fact, pelvic pain but it is often confused with sciatica as the pain affects a similar area. Using the following specific remedial exercises and preventative measures will easily distinguish sacro-iliac pain from sciatica. Although the exercises bring rapid relief, this is often short-lived so they should be repeated as often as you can. The reason for this is that the pelvis remains unstable throughout pregnancy in preparation for the birth. Once your baby is born, the symptoms will usually disappear.

If, however, you have tried the following suggestions and are still experiencing pain, you should see a physiotherapist, preferably one with a background in obstetrics.

Sacro-iliac pain is caused by the loosening of the pelvic joints, which in turn is caused by hormonal softening. This happens in order to widen the pelvic bony outlet and make the birth process easier. This hormonal softening can last from three to six months following the birth, but then disappears as the pelvis returns to normal. A simple description of the anatomy of the pelvis is helpful in understanding the nature of this discomfort.

The pelvis is a bony basin formed from the fusion of three bones, the sacrum and two iliac bones. This fusion creates three 'potential' joints known as the two sacro-iliac joints and the pubic symphysis. In the non-pregnant body these joints are potential or 'fused', which means that they cannot move. During pregnancy, however, your hormones destabilise this fusion and enable some degree of movement in all three joints. This is what causes the pain.

Management of sacro-iliac pain is based on limiting the movement in

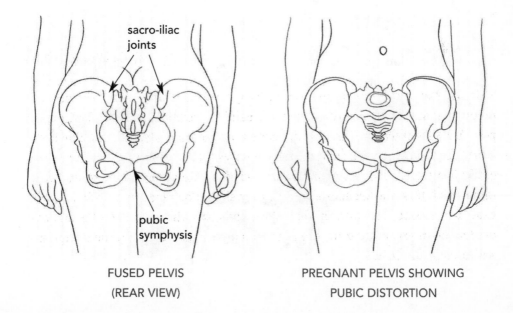

sacro-iliac joints

pubic symphysis

FUSED PELVIS
(REAR VIEW)

PREGNANT PELVIS SHOWING
PUBIC DISTORTION

these joints. It is possible to realign and almost restore the normal, or neutral, position of the joint using the self-mobilising techniques explained below.

These self-mobilising manoeuvres need to be repeated as often as required, sometimes 3 or 4 times a day.

Once the pain has been relieved the next step is to look at ways to prevent this 'destabilisation', and this too is quite simple. All you need to do is avoid any asymmetrical weight-bearing postures such as the relaxed 'standing-with-weight-on-one-leg' position, cross-leg sitting or pushing heavy objects with one leg.

How can we counteract the looseness in these joints? Since, under normal circumstances, we have no control over these joints, it is not surprising to find there are no specific individual muscles to act as stabilisers. However, the combined action of all the muscles that envelop the pelvis can provide significant support.

The pain of instability in these joints is often described as a 'stabbing' pain into the buttock or down the back of the thigh. It is easy to mistake as sciatica, but the pain of sciatica is more sustained, follows a line down the leg and can extend to beyond the knee.

MOVEMENTS TO SOOTHE PAINFUL SACRO-ILIAC JOINTS

The best position for these movements is lying down, but they can be done standing in situations where lying down is not possible such as while you are at work.

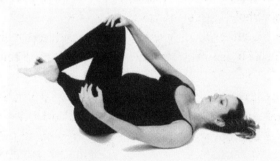

- As pictured on the previous page begin rolling your knees in a circular pattern, controlling the movement with your hands. Roll to massage the lower back and to identify the exact site of the pain.
- The pain will be situated a few centimetres either on the right or left of your lower back, this being the exact location of the sacro-iliac joint.
- Focus this rolling motion directly over the painful spot for about 10 revolutions. In most cases this eases the pain. If this is not the case, continue with the next movement.

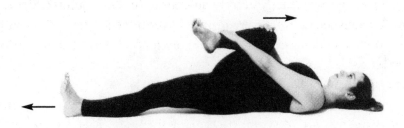

- Grip the leg of the painful side (as shown above), holding both your knee and ankle. Rotate your knee out to the side as much as you need to accommodate your bump.
- Straighten your other leg along the floor, pushing your heel away from you as hard as you can until you feel the relief at the back of your pelvis. This will mobilise the sacro-iliac joint and should relieve pain after a number of sustained pushes. Remember to engage your thigh muscles to lengthen the whole leg out of your hip socket.
- Repeat this on either side several times, breathing freely all the while. Don't be put off by an initial twinge of pain, as this is common before the pain eases.
- This movement can also be done the opposite way around. Hold the knee on the more comfortable side and stretch your other leg away.
- Either way is appropriate if the pain eases. You should always follow up

this movement with the bridging exercise on page 44 to test out the effectiveness of the pain relief.

You may achieve complete pain relief, but even if you only experience partial relief, this means that you are on the right track and it will only be a matter of repeating the procedure every few hours, together with implementing all the other preventative measures, before you are pain-free. This is a 'cranky, irritable joint' that is unstable in pregnancy and will remain unstable, needing to be realigned little and often on a daily basis, until your baby is born.

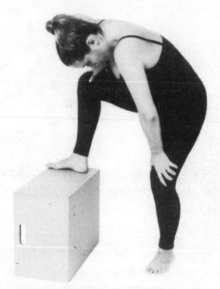

RELIEVING RIGHT SACRO-ILIAC PAIN

If you are at work and unable to lie down, you can still do the same manoeuvre. As shown above, stand with your right foot up on a chair. Vary both the position and height of your right knee by rotating it outwards and dropping your body weight between both knees until you find a position that relieves the pain. Feel the stretch in your right pelvis and buttock. Repeat to the left.

Follow this standing manoeuvre either with a squat (page 49) or a short bout of belly dancing in standing (page 27). Once again, this follow-up manoeuvre can be done discreetly, depending on your clothing, although if you work in an open-plan office environment, you may wish to find a more private place in which to do this.

PARTNER PULLING LEG

Having your partner pull your leg as shown below has a similar, if not better, effect.

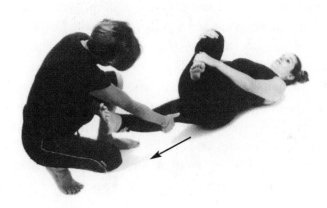

- While you are lying down, your partner, holding the back of your ankle and calf, pulls your leg towards them as shown above.
- Your partner should pull gently, only to the point at which you begin to feel a stretch. If they pull too hard, or too fast, you will feel a pinch as they release. They should also release gently.
- This movement should be repeated only 2 or 3 times on each leg.

MOVEMENTS TO AVOID

The following movements can aggravate sacro-iliac pain and should be avoided whenever possible:

- standing with your weight unevenly distributed between your legs;
- sitting with your legs crossed, that is, with most of your weight on one side of your pelvis;
- pushing heavy objects with your foot; and
- lying with all your weight on one side of the pelvis, even if you are propped up with pillows.

There are other movements that produce sacro-iliac pain, including walking on uneven surfaces and up and down stairs, rolling over in bed or, in some instances, walking of any kind and lifting – whether of babies, toddlers, baby paraphernalia or laundry baskets. Most of the above movements involve uneven weight distribution through the pelvis, which causes a skewing or twisting of the unstable bones in the pelvis. If you are careful, however, this can be avoided or minimised. This means being fastidious about distributing your weight evenly between both feet while deliberately bracing all the enveloping muscles of the pelvis. Lock up your pelvic joints with a deliberate squeeze of all the enveloping musculature. The pelvic floor exercises in Chapter 2 are designed to strengthen and increase your awareness of these muscles.

ADAPTATIONS TO EVERYDAY MOVEMENTS TO MINIMISE PAIN

When rolling over in bed, 'make like a mermaid' or keep your knees glued together and brace with all the muscles around the pelvis to give you extra stability as you move. You may find that rolling with a pillow gripped between the knees also reduces the pain.

WALKING WITH SACRO-ILIAC PAIN

Shorten your stride and squeeze with your buttock, tummy and pelvic floor muscles as you walk.

GETTING IN AND OUT OF THE CAR

Keep your knees together and lift both legs out at the same time. Squeeze with your buttock and tummy muscles and use your arms to lever your body weight up and out of the car.

GETTING UP OUT OF A CHAIR

Use your buttocks to squeeze around your pelvis and transfer your weight forwards through your feet *before* you lift. Use your leg muscles to help you rise.

PUBIC SYMPHYSIS PAIN

Situated in the front of the pelvis, the pubic symphysis, like the sacro-iliac, is once again not actually a joint but becomes one as a result of hormonal softening. It also has no specific muscle groups to stabilise it, which is why women are so vulnerable to this pain in pregnancy. This joint can become quite unstable, acutely painful and potentially most debilitating. Movements that exacerbate pain are: rolling over in bed, walking up slopes or stairs or, in severe cases, movement of any kind.

PAIN MANAGEMENT

The same management techniques apply as those for sacro-iliac pain, but it is imperative you avoid any asymmetrical weight-bearing postures that distort the pelvis. Some additional pain-management techniques include:

- **squatting** – paradoxically, stretching the joint in the squatting position gives a great deal of relief (see page 49).
- **walking pigeon-toed** – this turns on the pelvic muscles to act as a stronger brace around the pelvis. You will feel the buttock, inner thigh and outer thigh muscles contracting more strongly as you walk, which relieves the pain.
- **wearing a trochanter belt** – this compresses the pelvic joints and provides some degree of stability and pain relief. These belts can be purchased from surgical suppliers or pharmacies.
- **pillows in bed** – rolling over in bed can be more comfortable if you grip a pillow between your knees. Remember to brace with all the stabilising muscles around the pelvis before you move.
- **walking sticks** – additional support can help in some instances, as can taking small steps, avoiding long strides and wearing shoes with cushioned soles.
- **sitting on a ball** – this cushions your body weight, but only if you sit with your feet widely spaced and taking your weight through your feet.

ACHING BETWEEN THE SHOULDER BLADES

This is the thoracic spine and is notoriously stiff in women. Located at the level of the bra strap, part of the reason for this stiffness is, in my opinion, our reluctance to stick our chests out, which is what happens when this part of the spine is postured correctly. Many women understandably, have a tendency to be a little conservative about posturing the spine at this level, especially during pregnancy when breast size can change quite significantly. The sheer weight of the breasts pulls down on the thoracic or upper back, which results in a deeper curve or humped posture. Another possible cause of pain could be the subconscious postural adjustments or stiffening of the thoracic spine you make to accommodate your growing baby.

Some women experience discomfort in this area for the first time in pregnancy, for others, their pregnancy may have exacerbated a chronic

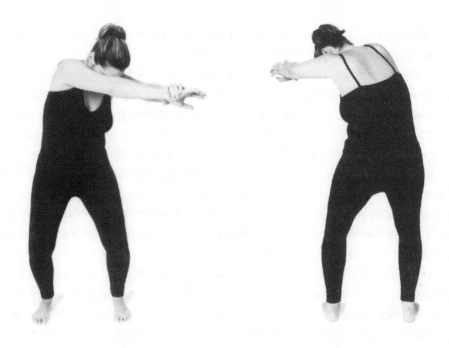

low-grade discomfort. In either case, mobilising the spine will give immediate relief. The discomfort or pain may require daily management, however, which is not unreasonable considering the problem may have been there for years. Stiff thoracic spines need ongoing and, indeed, lifelong mobilising.

The best exercises for mobilising your thoracic spine are:

- Spinal twist in standing
- Draping in standing
- Side stretch on ball
- Chin draping in standing
- Chin draping

A BURNING FEELING AROUND THE RIB CAGE

This can be attributed to one of two things. One may be the discomfort felt where the abdominal muscles meet the ribs. As your baby grows and stretches your abdominal wall, these points of insertion are placed under considerable strain, and this may cause the pain. Surprisingly, adding a gentle stretch to the affected area often relieves pain.

The other possibility may be pain referred from the thoracic spine. As we have seen, this part of the spine becomes very stiff in pregnancy as women brace or hold themselves too erect in order to create more space for breathing. Thoracic rotations will reverse both the stiffness as well as the referred pain, and the best exercises for this are listed below.

As we have seen above, if you have an underlying predisposition to stiffness in the thoracic spine, this will become worse during your pregnancy. If you happen to be one of those who are stiff, treat this as the perfect opportunity to make lifelong changes and keep your spine flexible for life.

The best exercises for alleviating that burning feeling around the rib cage are:

- Draping
- Chin draping
- Spinal twist in standing
- Double posture challenge – side bend
- Rotations in side lying

COCCYX PAIN

Your coccyx is situated at the base of your spine and can become painful either during your pregnancy or after your baby is born. It is also called the tail bone, and can easily be felt just above your anus. Sitting is, obviously, the most provocative position, but this can be easily remedied by modifying how you sit. Practising your pelvic floor contractions can also ease the discomfort, particularly after the birth. This is because the pelvic floor muscles attach directly to the coccyx and muscular activity reduces any dragging sensation or pull at the point of attachment. See pages 16–18, for a full description of pelvic floor exercises and how to do them.

SITTING COMFORTABLY WITH COCCYX PAIN

Good sitting posture significantly reduces the pressure on your coccyx. The weight of your body should be focused on the sitting bones to the front, while your thighs and feet are also taking some of the burden. Poor posture will result in your pelvis rolling backwards. This will shift your body weight away from the thighs and feet, directly on to your coccyx. To keep the pelvis rolled forwards your coccyx, your spine *must* be in neutral, which requires a strong, flexible back and strong tummy muscles.

REMEDIAL MEASURES

If, after checking and correcting your sitting posture, you are still experiencing pain, you can try some or all of the following:

- Ice or heat therapy in the lying-down position. Use ice in the form of a frozen peri-pad, or disposable nappy, placed between the buttocks as close to the pain as possible. A soft hot pack can also relieve pain and a good homemade version is a damp towel, heated in the microwave and placed over the painful area.
- Sit on a ball. Team this with perfect sitting posture and it will significantly reduce the pressure on your coccyx and pain. If you are still experiencing pain a few weeks after the birth, use the ball to belly dance or pelvic roll (sitting directly on the coccyx), which will gently massage the painful area.
- Once again, be diligent about your pelvic floor exercises and try belly dancing in all the positions.

HEATING WET TOWELS IN THE MICROWAVE

These hot packs can be used for a variety of reasons, including breast engorgement, or lower back pain. Just fold the towel to the appropriate shape.

- Soak a small towel in water and wring it out completely.
- Fold it to the desired shape, then place it in a microwave-safe plastic bag and microwave on High for about 90 seconds or until it is the required heat.
- Dampen a tea-towel with cool water and wring it out. Remove the heated towel from the plastic bag and place it on to the tea-towel. Wrap the heated towel in the tea-towel.
- Before use, test the wrapped towel on the inner side of your forearm to be sure it is not too hot. The tea-towel will absorb any steam and prevent you being burned.

ROUND LIGAMENT PAIN

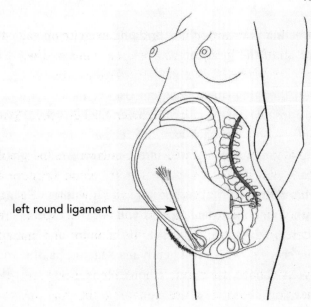

left round ligament

This presents as an acute pain in the groin or lower abdomen. It can be a short, stabbing pain or may be sustained over a period of time. There are two round ligaments, one on either side of the uterus. (The left round ligament is shown on the previous page.) They work together to stabilise the uterus within the abdominal cavity. Once your baby has grown to the point where your uterus begins to reach upwards into the abdominal cavity, these ligaments are placed under increasing strain to the point where certain movements trigger pain. This is caused by tiny muscle fibres within the ligaments going into spasm as they are overstretched.

A good way to prevent the muscle fibres going into spasm is to brace around your uterus with your tummy muscles. This stabilises the uterus and reduces strain on the ligaments, so preventing the muscle fibres from going into spasm.

This bracing will help prevent round ligament pain during activities as varied as rapid walking, climbing stairs or simply rolling over in bed.

REVERSING PERSISTENT PAIN

If the pain persists beyond a few minutes, try the bridging exercise on page 43. Sustain the hold for a few minutes if you can or use your hands or pillows to support your pelvis. This eases out the spasm and reduces the pain.

SWOLLEN HANDS AND FEET (OEDEMA)

While this is usually an innocuous condition which responds well to the simple remedies suggested below, you should check that your blood pressure is normal. Swelling or oedema caused by fluid retention can sometimes be a sign of high blood pressure, and a potentially dangerous condition known as pre-eclampsia. If this is the case, your doctor will carefully monitor and manage your condition.

During pregnancy, you have an extra unit of blood being pumped around your system and your hormones are softening the tiny muscles supporting your blood vessels. This could be part of the explanation why some women have oedema or fluid retention in the hands and feet.

Fluid in the hands is sometimes called carpal tunnel syndrome. Its symptoms are eased by elevating and resting the whole arm on a pillow above shoulder level, massage and ice packs. It is also helpful to do arm pumping and shoulder exercises. Some women find that using a splint to support the wrist while they are sleeping is effective in reducing pain and, indeed, some continue to use the splint during the day. If the problem exists in only one hand, you should avoid sleeping on the affected side. This condition also produces a loss of dexterity, with many women complaining that they are 'dropping things all the time'. Physiotherapists can use therapeutic ultrasound when the condition becomes acute.

Exercising the whole of the upper limb, as in the push-up exercise on page 38 is recommended as this produces a pumping effect on all the muscles in the arm and reduces the fluid retention.

One of the most effective remedies for swollen feet is to elevate them just a few centimetres above the level of the heart. This is easily done by lying down and placing your legs on pillows. This gives only temporary relief, however, and will need to be done little and often. Wearing support stockings is very successful in controlling oedema. Maintaining an exercise program will strengthen your leg muscles and reduce the swelling.

Dietary influences are also directly linked to fluid retention, especially consuming too much salt. Keep your salt intake under control and remember that there are many natural diuretics that may help with fluid retention, including celery, green apples, parsley, nectarines, water melon and dandelion. You should be drinking at least two litres of water a day.

RESTLESS LEGS

This is a common complaint in pregnancy which can leave you feeling like you are running a nightly marathon race in bed as you search incessantly for the comfortable position. Try placing a couple of very large European pillows under your legs or even wrap a spare doona around your legs. The point of this is to stabilise your legs long enough to allow your torso or trunk muscles to relax. Your restless legs may also be due to calf muscle congestion, which can be alleviated by doing some leg pumping exercises in bed. Try a few minutes of vigorous pumping of the ankles up, down, round and round.

VARICOSE VEINS

Varicose veins are another fairly common condition associated with pregnancy, especially in second-time mums. Venous congestion is caused by the baby's presence in the pelvis, where it impedes the return of blood back up from the legs to the heart. Of course, it is not a true impediment, but its presence compounds the effects of the hormonal softening of the blood vessels. Slowing the blood flow can produce the congestion in the legs that results in varicose veins.

Strong leg muscles compensate for this sluggish blood flow as will the wearing of support stockings. These come in varying strengths and need professional fitting, either at a chemist or surgical supplier. Elevating your legs is very effective. You must support the whole leg with pillows and be very careful not to add any additional pressure at any point along the leg, especially at the level of the affected veins.

LEG CRAMPS

All of the above may occur in combination with leg cramps and all the remedies suggested above are also effective with cramping. The most effective form of prevention of cramping is to have strong, elastic muscles and to stretch the muscles that cramp before you go to bed.

ACHING FEET

As we have discussed already, some problems are not caused by, but exacerbated in pregnancy. Aching feet can be attributed both to weight gain and hormonal softening, but usually only occur in conjunction with an underlying weakness such as dropped arches or poor pedal posture. It is important to remember that posture correction applies not only to the spine, but to the feet as well.

Your foot pain may be caused by falling arches. You can try to reinstate your arch by lifting the inside of your foot and bearing more of your weight on the outside of the foot. Bracing the small muscles in the foot creates a good support structure for these arches, then the long muscles at the front of the shin will correct the posture of the whole of the ankle. In other words you need to be proactive about bracing your foot muscles with every step you take. If this all sounds too confusing, your physiotherapist can quickly teach you how to correct your foot posture.

CONCLUSION

Now that you have a few strategies to help ease the musculoskeletal discomforts common in pregnancy, I hope that you feel a sense of reassurance that there is a lot that you can do to make your pregnancy as comfortable and manageable as possible.

While pregnancy can be a somewhat mystical time for many new mums there is nothing illogical or extraordinary about the changes that are taking place in your body, or their accompanying symptoms. The logical part is the reality of the effects of carrying the load of your rapidly growing baby. It sure gets heavy some days. And all of this is occurring as your body softens in preparation for birth. It is no wonder that pregnant women feel more comfortable when they are fit and strong.

What I do know from the women in my classes is that the fitter and stronger you are both before your pregnancy and the stronger you become during your pregnancy, the more comfortable and confident you will be in your pregnancy.

I hope that the exercises and pain-management techniques in this book will help you to power through your pregnancy – good luck!